SPRINGHOUSE
CLINICAL
ROTATION

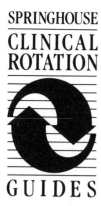

GUIDES

SURGICAL NURSING

Mary Jane Evans, RN, BSN, CCRN
Mary Ann Black, RN, PhD, CCRN

Springhouse Corporation
Springhouse, Pennsylvania

MW00463970

Staff For This Volume

Executive Director, Editorial
Stanley Loeb

Executive Director, Creative Services
Jean Robinson

Director of Trade and Textbooks
Minnie B. Rose, RN, BSN, MEd

Art Director
John Hubbard

Editorial Manager
Kevin Law

Editors
Bernadette Glenn (acquisitions associate), Diane Labus, David Moreau

Copy Editor
Keith de Pinho

Designers
Stephanie Peters (associate art director), Julie Carleton Barlow

Art Production
Robert Perry (manager), Anna Brindisi, Donald Knauss, Catherine Mace, Robert Wieder

Typography
David Kosten (manager), Diane Paluba (assistant manager), Joyce Rossi Biletz, Brenda Mayer, Robin Rantz, Brent Rinedoller, Valerie Rosenberger

Manufacturing
Deborah Meiris (manager), T.A. Landis, Jennifer Suter

Project Coordination
Aline S. Miller (manager), Maura C. Murphy

Library of Congress Cataloging-in-Publication Data
Evans, Mary Jane R.
  Surgical nursing/Mary Jane Evans, Mary Ann Black.
    p. cm.—(Springhouse clinical rotation guides)
  Bibliography: p.
  Includes index.
  1. Surgical nursing—Handbooks, manuals, etc. I. Black, Mary Ann. II. Title. III. Series: Clinical rotation guides.
  [DNLM: 1. Surgical Nursing. WY 161 E92s]
RD99.24.E93 1990
610.73′677—dc20
DNLM/DLC
for Library of Congress   89-10092
ISBN 0-87434-207-4   CIP

To my husband, Corey H. Evans, MD,
for his unfailing emotional support throughout the series.
To my children, Christopher and Michael,
for their patience and love.
And to Mary Ann Black, RN, PhD, for her friendship and profes-
sional assistance
beyond the call of duty.
MJE

This book is dedicated to my mother, with love.
MAB

Table of Contents

Special Acknowledgment

The series consulting editor wishes to thank Florida Hospital, Orlando, Florida, owned and operated by the Adventist Health System, for the services and support that made this series possible.

Series Consulting Editor
Mary Jane Evans, RN, BSN, CCRN
Independent Consultant for Nursing Education

Clinical Consultants
Corey H. Evans, MD
Associate Director
Family Practice Residency
Florida Hospital
Orlando, Fla.

Dennis G. Ross, RN, MSN, MAE, CNOR
Associate Professor of Nursing
Castleton State College
Castleton, Vt.

Advisory Board

Surgical Nursing

Diane Sadler Benson, RN, MEd, MS
Nurse Specialist and Educator in Private Practice
Benson-Sadler Enterprises, Ltd.
Eureka, Calif.

Marie Scott Brown, RN, PNP, PhD
Professor of Family Nursing
School of Nursing
Oregon Health Science University
Portland, Ore.

Lillian S. Brunner, RN, MSN, ScD, LittD, FAAN
Nurse-Author
Brunner Associates, Inc.
Berwyn, Pa.

Joanne V. Hickey, RN, BSN, MSN, MA, PhD
Professor of Nursing and Independent Consultant
in Neuroscience Nursing
Community College of Rhode Island
Warwick, R.I.

Nancy M. Holloway, RN, MSN, CCRN, CEN
Critical Care and Emergency Consultant
Nancy Holloway Associates
Oakland, Calif.

Celestine B. Mason, RN, BSN, MA
Nursing Care Consultant
Good Samaritan Hospital
Puyallup, Wash.;
Former Associate Professor of Nursing
Pacific Lutheran University
Tacoma, Wash.

Dennis G. Ross, RN, MSN, MAE, CNOR
Associate Professor of Nursing
Castleton State College
Castleton, Vt.

Carol E. Smith, RN, PhD
Professor, School of Nursing
University of Kansas
Kansas City, Kan.

Preface

This book, developed as a supplementary aid, will assist the student in planning and implementing care of the surgical patient in the clinical setting. It in no way substitutes for an in-depth study of surgical patient care; rather, it provides quick access to information useful to nursing students on surgical rotations.

Within this book, the student will find clinical instruction on:
• obtaining a nursing history and performing a physical assessment on the preoperative patient
• preoperative care and patient teaching
• postoperative care and complications frequently associated with recovery
• wound and burn care, including techniques for dressings and suture removal
• nursing diagnoses and interventions associated with the perioperative period
• techniques of common surgeries, including illustrations and descriptions of common operative procedures
• use of equipment, tubes, and drains
• surgical emergencies
• medications frequently used in surgical areas.

1 Admitting the Surgical Patient

The data you obtain from the patient's admission history and physical assessment, along with data from the immediate preoperative assessment, establish a baseline for postoperative evaluation. This information also allows you to implement preventive and precautionary interventions before surgery for patients who potentially are at high risk.

For example, assessing the effects of anesthesia and immobility on the lungs postoperatively would be extremely difficult if you had no idea of the patient's condition preoperatively. However, if you knew the patient was a smoker and had signs of lung congestion before surgery, you could support his efforts to stop smoking, assess his current respiratory status, and intervene with measures to improve his respiratory status before surgery. Immediately before the patient is moved to the operating room, you could assess and document his respiratory status again to allow for a baseline comparison postoperatively.

☐ Patient history

The first step of the admission assessment involves taking the patient history. Many hospitals have patient admission history sheets to help nurses gather this information systematically. Some hospitals use self-history forms designed for the patient to complete at his convenience after admission. If your hospital uses this type of form, review the first few questions with the patient. If he appears to be in no discomfort and can read and understand the questions, allow him to complete the form.

Keep in mind that the preoperative patient's anxiety level usually is extremely high and that even the simplest question may appear confusing. Let the patient know you'll be available to answer any questions he does not understand. Also remember that a written questionnaire is no substitute for a nursing history. Discuss any questions dealing with allergies, present or past illnesses (such as diabetes), or any problems that pose potential risk directly with the patient. Use self-history forms for supplemental information only.

General information

When taking the patient history, obtain the following general information as circumstances permit:
• biographic information (such as name, age, occupation, and religion)

• chief complaint (the main problem that caused the patient to seek help)
• present illness and health status (including any medications, complaints, or symptoms)
• previous history of illness (including hospitalizations, surgeries, and chronic illnesses)
• family history of illness (such as diabetes mellitus, heart disease, or anemia)
• review of body systems (including physiologic, psychological, and social implications)
• nutritional data (including current nutritional status, daily caloric intake, and food preferences).

Keep in mind that, in some situations, you may find it impossible to complete the entire nursing history in just one session. You may be interrupted by doctors or scheduled diagnostic tests, or the patient may be in too much discomfort to cooperate with your questioning. In such cases, prioritize your questions to obtain the information pertinent to the patient's immediate needs. For example, if the patient is in pain, you may need to evaluate the pain or chief complaint and intervene before continuing the history taking. Also, if the patient is taking special medications, you would need to know the types of medication, why he was taking them, and whether he brought any medication to the hospital.

Additional preoperative information
Besides the data you collect during the general patient history, you'll need to pay particular attention to the following information, which is associated with increased surgical risk.

Pulmonary function
Find out the following:
• Is the patient a smoker? If so, how many packs has he smoked per day and for how many years?
Rationale: Smoking increases postoperative respiratory complications and should be stopped 1 week before surgery, if possible. Smoking decreases the amount of functional hemoglobin available and impairs oxygen delivery to the tissues.
• Does the patient have any allergic conditions, such as asthma or hay fever? Has he had anesthesia-related problems with any previous surgeries?
Rationale: This may affect the choice of anesthetic agents.
• Does the patient have a chronic obstructive pulmonary disease? (This includes chronic bronchitis, emphysema, asthma, and bronchiectasis.) Has he had a recent acute upper respiratory infection?
Rationale: These disorders increase the risk of postoperative respiratory complications and may require preoperative interven-

tions to correct electrolyte imbalances (respiratory acidosis), prevent postoperative respiratory infection, or remove excess sputum.
• Is the patient immobile or on sedatives? Does he have pain that prevents full lung expansion?
Rationale: All of these factors contribute to hypoventilation, which can cause preoperative electrolyte problems and postoperative respiratory complications.
• If the patient has a respiratory disorder, were baseline arterial blood gas (ABG) levels obtained? If so, what are the levels?
Rationale: ABG levels are obtained preoperatively if the patient has respiratory problems or if cardiovascular surgery is scheduled. Normal values are as follows:

pH: 7.35 to 7.45
$PaCO_2$: 35 to 45 mm Hg
HCO_3^-: 22 to 26 mEq/liter
PaO_2: 80 to 100 mm Hg
Oxygen saturation: 94% to 100%.

Cardiovascular function

Determine the following:
• Does the patient have a history of cardiovascular disease?
Rationale: Anything that causes the heart to pump ineffectively, resulting in reduced cardiac output, places the patient at risk for developing both preoperative and postoperative complications. Inadequate blood volume and ineffective vasoconstriction also increase surgical risk.

The degree of risk depends on the extent of the cardiovascular problem. Sometimes, such a problem may contraindicate elective surgery. For example, elective surgery usually is postponed for patients with angina pectoris, unstable angina, severe aortic stenosis, atrioventricular block (high, with syncopal symptoms), severe hypertension, or cardiac failure, and for those suffering a myocardial infarction within the previous 6 months.
• Does the patient complain of symptoms or problems associated with compromised cardiovascular function, including shortness of breath, lung congestion, edema, abdominal (liver) tenderness, hypertension, and palpitations, or chest pain at rest or on exertion? Does he have symptoms of peripheral vascular disease, such as coolness, pain, claudication, numbness or tingling, edema, or diminished or absent pulses in an extremity?
Rationale: Such a patient requires further evaluation by a doctor before surgery. Presurgical intervention depends on the extent of the disorder. Sometimes, mild or asymptomatic cardiac problems are diagnosed initially during a preoperative examination. Pay close attention to assessing the more subtle symptoms of cardiovascular disease.

Neurologic function

Find out the following:

• Does the patient have any history of neurologic disorders, such as epilepsy, Parkinson's disease, multiple sclerosis, or myasthenia gravis?

Rationale: Such a patient requires special precautions pertaining to preoperative use of long-term medications. Check with the patient's doctor or anesthesiologist.

• Is the patient taking antidepressants, sedatives, neuroleptics, antianxiety agents, or other medications that directly affect the nervous system?

Rationale: Such a patient requires preoperative changes in medication or anesthesia.

• Does the patient display signs and symptoms suggesting significant neurologic problems, including persistent headache, numbness or tingling in an extremity, tremors or weakness in an extremity, unsteady gait, confusion, and loss of memory?

Rationale: A patient with an apparent or suspected neurologic deficit is at risk for surgical complications. The patient's postoperative neurologic status is compared with preoperative assessment data and the admission history to evaluate recovery. Report any neurologic signs and symptoms to the doctor.

Renal function

Determine the following:

• Does the patient have any complaints associated with kidney or bladder infection? Urinary frequency or urgency? Burning on urination? Blood in the urine (hematuria)? Fever? Back, flank, or suprapubic pain?

Rationale: A patient with signs and symptoms of urinary or kidney infection needs more extensive preoperative evaluation. If renal function is severely compromised by infection, the stress of surgery can precipitate renal failure. Laboratory data associated with renal problems include abnormal urinalysis results and abnormal blood urea nitrogen (BUN) and creatinine levels.

• Does the patient have chronic renal disease?

Rationale: With decreased renal function, the patient has a mass of nonfunctioning renal tissue. The remaining functional renal tissue maintains homeostasis of the extracellular fluid, leaving little functional tissue to deal with the acute stressors of the perioperative period and thereby increasing the risk of acute renal failure. Be sure to monitor the patient's BUN and creatinine levels when available.

Immunologic function

Find out the following:

• Is the patient allergic to any foods, medications, soaps, or depilatories?

Rationale: Some allergic reactions to medication can be fatal; some can be serious enough to permanently damage vital organs, such as the kidneys. Be sure to question the patient about any history of hypersensitivity reactions. Note any allergies to shellfish and seafood and to soaps containing iodine or hexachlorophene. A skin reaction to a presurgical scrub can result in postponement of the surgical procedure.

Endocrine function

Determine the following:
• Is the patient diabetic?
Rationale: Diabetes mellitus puts the patient at risk for delayed wound healing, postoperative surgical infection, and hyperglycemic or hypoglycemic episodes throughout the perioperative period. A diabetic patient requires special interventions to control the disorder throughout the perioperative period.
• Is the patient taking steroids or has he been treated with steroid medications within the past year?
Rationale: Steroid use can cause adrenocortical insufficiency. Normally, the adrenal glands produce about 25 mg of cortisol daily; however, during the stress of surgery, the adrenal glands may secrete 250 to 300 mg daily. Steroid use also can suppress production of cortisol, sometimes for weeks or months after the patient is weaned from the medication. Long-term, high-dose use may lead to adrenal atrophy, requiring special tests to evaluate adrenal function before surgery.
• Is the patient an alcoholic?
Rationale: Chronic alcoholism suppresses the adrenocortical response to operative stress. If the patient does not admit to drinking heavily and you are concerned that he might be an alcoholic, share these concerns with the patient's surgeon. Keep in mind that alcoholic patients are at risk for delirium tremens with withdrawal.

Hematologic function

Determine the following:
• Does the patient have a bleeding disorder?
Rationale: Abnormal coagulation factors increase the patient's risk of hemorrhage, hematoma formation, delayed wound healing, and infection.
• Does the patient have symptoms suggesting a possible bleeding disorder? These may include a history of easy bruising, nosebleeds, excessive use of aspirin, and previous use of anticoagulants or other drugs with an anticoagulant action. Check the patient's hematologic profile for abnormal bleeding time, platelet count, prothrombin time, or partial thromboplastin time.

Rationale: Preoperative diagnosis of a bleeding disorder can avert serious hemorrhagic complications. Report any of the suspicious findings listed above to your instructor.

Infection

Find out about the following:
• Does the patient have an upper or lower respiratory infection?
Rationale: Anesthesia produces increased bronchial secretions besides the congestion already present in cases of respiratory infection. This has a profound effect on ventilation in the postoperative patient.
• Does the patient have an infection near the surgical site or the lymphatic vessels that drain that area?
Rationale: If the patient has such an infection, notify the doctor immediately, as this may be reason enough to postpone surgery. The surgical incision site should be free from contamination and supplied with adequate lymphatic drainage to ensure proper wound healing. Report any rashes, carbuncles, or any type of skin irritation.
• Does the patient have any other signs and symptoms suggesting underlying infection, including fever, malaise and flulike complaints, symptoms of urinary tract infections, or sneezing and signs of allergy or upper respiratory infection?
Rationale: Osteomyelitis, chronic inflammatory diseases, and inflammation decrease the stress response and decrease hematopoiesis.

Gastrointestinal (GI) function

Ask about the following:
• Does the patient complain of nausea, vomiting, diarrhea, constipation, present or previous ulcer disease, inflammatory bowel disorders, or diverticular disease? Has he ever experienced bleeding from the upper or lower GI tract?
Rationale: Anesthesia and preoperative pain medications affect GI function. You will need to obtain an adequate history for postoperative comparison.

☐ Physical assessment

You'll need to perform a preoperative physical assessment to uncover any physiologic factors that place the patient at risk for postoperative complications and to establish a baseline of the patient's present health status for reference during the postoperative recovery period. To perform a complete assessment, you'll use the techniques of inspection, palpation, percussion, and auscultation. Begin as soon as possible after the patient is admitted to the surgical unit.

During your assessment, be sure to note the following data, which may help reduce the patient's surgical risk.

Nutritional status

Assess the following:
• What is the patient's apparent nutritional state? Does he appear cachectic or obese?
• Does he have an eating behavior disorder, such as anorexia or bulimia? (Signs and symptoms include bruising of the knuckles of the dominant hand from excessive induced vomiting, fatigue, and hypertrophied salivary glands.)
• Is the patient's diet nutritionally adequate? (Ask the patient what he normally eats daily.)
• Does the patient follow dietary restrictions if he is on a special diet?
Rationale: Postoperative wound healing and homeostasis depend upon the patient's nutritional status.

Vital signs

Take vital signs and report any abnormal findings.
Rationale: Abnormal vital signs may signal the possibility of infection or respiratory or cardiovascular problems that may warrant further investigation before surgery.

Mental and neurologic status

Determine whether the patient is oriented, and assess his level of consciousness. Perform a thorough neurologic examination and record your findings. Notify the doctor of any abnormal signs and symptoms.
Rationale: Postoperative neurologic and behavioral changes can result from the effects of anesthetics, analgesics, or sedatives on the central nervous system—especially in elderly patients. A baseline preoperative neurologic assessment is essential.

Skin

Assess for evidence of mottling, edema, coolness, decreased capillary refill, diminished or absent pulses, cyanosis, and other signs of poor perfusion. Note any lesions, infections, or rashes in the area surrounding the surgical site.
Rationale: Signs of perfusion problems place the patient at risk for postoperative complications and indicate a need for further investigation by a doctor. Lesions, inflammation, or rashes around the proposed surgical site may warrant postponement of surgery. Report any such skin changes promptly.

Pulmonary status

Any disease or disorder that involves some degree of airway obstruction places the patient at risk for developing postoperative pulmonary complications. Acute respiratory conditions usually involve such infections as pharyngitis, flu, pneumonias, and colds. In such cases, the patient usually is started on antibiotic therapy, and elective surgery is postponed until the acute episode resolves.

Chronic lung diseases, such as emphysema, asthma, bronchitis, and bronchiectasis, present an even greater surgical risk. A patient with such a disorder may be hospitalized for at least 1 week and treated with antibiotics, nebulized bronchodilators, intermittent positive-pressure ventilation, and respiratory exercises. Because postoperative pulmonary complications are common and possibly quite serious, you'll want to give special attention to the preoperative respiratory assessment.

Have the patient undress from the waist up or wear a hospital gown with a front opening. With the patient seated on the side of the bed, examine him for the following:

Neck and chest wall. Is the chest normally shaped? Does breathing cause the chest to rise symmetrically? Do you notice any intercostal retractions (indentations of the skin between the ribs caused by labored respiration)? Does he use accessory muscles (neck, circumoral) in breathing?
Rationale: Asymmetrical chest movement suggests possible pneumothorax or pain that restricts movement of the rib cage and impairs ventilation. The use of accessory muscles or intercostal retractions (or both) indicates abnormally labored respirations, usually from chronic obstructive or restrictive lung disease.

An abnormally shaped chest, such as the barrel chest seen in patients with emphysema, can indicate chronic lung disease. Severe spinal deformities, such as scoliosis, can compromise lung expansion and ventilation. All of these findings place the patient at risk for postoperative complications.

Tachypnea. Is the patient's respiratory rate greater than 25 respirations per minute?
Rationale: The patient may be compensating for his inability to breathe deeply by breathing more rapidly. Tachypnea, which may result from restrictive or obstructive lung problems, is an extremely important physical finding. Be sure to alert the doctor, who will further evaluate the patient before surgery to determine the cause.

Increased fremitus. Use the top portion of your palm to palpate along the anterior and posterior intercostal spaces while the patient repeats the word "ninety-nine." Note whether you can feel excessive vibrations through the chest wall.
Rationale: Increased fremitus may point to consolidation of lung tissue (increased lung density resulting from retained fluid, exudate, or lung debris), a significant sign that may indicate increased risk of postoperative atelectasis or alveolar collapse.

Lung fields. Place the diaphragm of your stethoscope over the intercostal spaces, starting at the top of the lungs and working toward the lung bases. Auscultate anteriorly and posteriorly. Listen for the following abnormal sounds, which may indicate pulmonary problems:
• crackles—discontinuous crackling sounds heard over the lung fields of smaller airways
• wheezes—continuous high-pitched musical sounds heard over the lung fields
• rhonchi—bubbling sounds heard over the major airways and their branches.

These abnormal sounds reflect the amount and quality (dry or moist) of fluid in the airways as well as the condition of the alveoli and lung tissue. Be sure to record your findings and to mention the lung field over which you heard the abnormal sound (see *Surface anatomy and lung fields,* page 10). Also be sure to evaluate and record any abnormal (adventitious) breath sounds you note during auscultation (see *Assessing abnormal breath sounds,* page 11).

Use percussion to compare each side of the chest at each intercostal space. Starting at the top of the lungs, work your way toward the lung bases, alternating from one side of the chest to the other as you listen for the following abnormal sounds (percuss both the anterior and posterior lung fields):
• hyperresonance—a low-pitched and booming sound, associated with such diseases as emphysema, in which air becomes trapped in the lung (Diminished or absent resonance results from an absence of air in a section of the lung from the collapse of alveoli.)
• dullness—a thudlike sound (usually heard over the liver), possibly indicating consolidation or dense lung tissue from fluid or a neoplasm
• flatness—an extremely dull sound with no noticeable resonance; usually heard over bones (sternum), flatness is associated with disorders that produce atelectasis.

Cardiovascular status

Because patients with even minor or asymptomatic cardiac disorders may be subject to myocardial ischemia, cardiac failure, and serious dysrhythmias during the operative and postoperative period, all preoperative patients require a thorough cardiovascular assessment.

Any condition severe enough to mildly impair cardiac output warrants further investigation by a doctor. Preexisting conditions most commonly associated with increased surgical risk include cardiac failure, coronary heart disease (with a history of myocardial infarction or angina pectoris), major dysrhythmias, valvular heart disease, and congenital heart disease.

SURFACE ANATOMY AND LUNG FIELDS

Use your knowledge of surface anatomy to visualize your patient's lung fields during a respiratory assessment. The illustrations below show the relationship of bony landmarks and lung position.

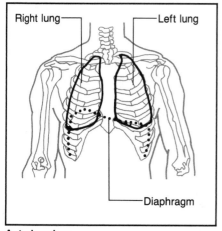

Anterior view

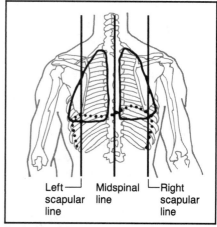

Posterior view

When assessing a patient's cardiovascular status, note the following signs and symptoms associated with compromised cardiac output:
• fatigue on exertion or at rest
• shortness of breath
• central nervous system changes
• syncope
• signs of cardiac failure, including:
　—decreased urine output
　—decreased blood pressure
　—jugular vein distention
　—basilar crackles
　—displaced point of maximal impulse (PMI)
　—sustained apical pulse
　—weight change with edema (greater than 2 lb/day)
　—irregular pulse rate or rhythm
　—dysrhythmias.

Heart sounds. If you have learned the technique of auscultation, listen to the patient's heart and confirm any abnormal findings with your instructor or an experienced nurse. Report any abnormal sounds, rubs, or murmurs immediately (see *Implications of abnormal heart sounds and murmurs,* page 12).

ASSESSING ABNORMAL BREATH SOUNDS

Percuss and auscultate your patient's chest. The chart below will help you identify abnormal breath sounds associated with respiratory disorders.

Disorder	Percussion	Abnormal breath sounds
Consolidation	Dull	Fine crackles early; coarse crackles later
Atelectasis	Dull	Fine crackles early; coarse crackles later
Pleural effusion or empyema	Dull to absent	Pleural friction rub
Pneumothorax	Normal or hyperresonant	Fine crackles when fluid is present
Acute or chronic bronchitis	Normal	Rhonchi; coarse crackles
Bronchial asthma	Normal or hyperresonant	Wheezes
Pulmonary edema	Normal or dull	Coarse crackles

If you have not yet learned how to auscultate the heart, use the following guidelines for a general assessment:

• Using the diaphragm of your stethoscope, auscultate the area over the fifth intercostal space at the midclavicular line. Determine the patient's apical pulse rate. Note any rates below 60 beats/minute or above 100 beats/minute or any irregularities in rhythm.

• Palpate for the PMI, noting any displacement to the left of the midclavicular line.

• If the apical pulse is irregular, obtain an apical-radial pulse. (Two nurses—one palpating the radial pulse, one auscultating the apical pulse—count the heart rate for 1 minute using the same watch.) Record any pulse deficit—an apical increase of more than 10 beats over the radial (peripheral) pulse rate. Dysrhythmias may be responsible for this decrease in peripheral perfusion.

• Listen over the apex for the "lub-dub" sound of a normal cardiac cycle. "Lub," the first heart sound (S_1), represents the systolic phase of the cardiac cycle. "Dub," the second heart sound (S_2), represents the diastolic phase of the cycle. Be sure to report any extra sounds, vibrations, rasping, or friction noises.

Peripheral vascular disease. Immediately report any evidence of peripheral vascular disease not previously noted in the patient's chart. Signs and symptoms include:

• diminished or absent peripheral pulses or bruits (vibratory turbulence heard over a vessel) on auscultation (popliteal and femoral)

IMPLICATIONS OF ABNORMAL HEART SOUNDS AND MURMURS

Abnormal heart sounds	Timing	Possible causes
Accentuated S_1	Beginning of systole	• Hyperkinetic disorders, such as fever or mitral stenosis
Diminished S_1	Beginning of systole	• Mitral regurgitation • Severe mitral regurgitation with calcified immobile valve • Heart block
Accentuated S_2	End of systole	• Pulmonary or systemic hypertension
Diminished or inaudible S_2	End of systole	• Aortic or pulmonary stenosis
Persistent S_2 split	End of systole	• Delayed closure of the pulmonic valve, usually from overfilling of the right ventricle causing prolonged systolic ejection time
Persistent S_2 split that widens during inspiration	End of systole	• Pulmonic valve stenosis • Atrial ventricular septal defect • Right bundle branch block
Reversed or paradoxical S_2 split that appears in expiration and disappears in inspiration	End of systole	• Delayed ventricular stimulation (left bundle branch block or prolonged left ventricular ejection time)
S_3 (ventricular gallop)	Early diastole	• Normal in children and young adults • Overdistention of ventricle in rapid-filling segment of diastole (mitral insufficiency or ventricular failure)
S_4 (atrial gallop or presystolic extra sound)	Late diastole	• Forceful atrial contraction from resistance to ventricular filling late in diastole (left ventricular hypertrophy, pulmonary stenosis, hypertension, coronary artery disease, and aortic stenosis)
Pericardial friction rub (grating or leathery sound at left sternal border; usually muffled, high-pitched, and transient)	Throughout systole and diastole	• Pericardial inflammation

• asymmetry of pulse quality, intensity, or amplitude
• pain in the legs (calves) and feet relieved by rest (claudication)
• absence of hair from midcalf to the ankle with dry, shiny skin
• varicose veins
• temperature changes
• poor capillary refill time
• edema
• evidence of deep vein thrombosis or inflammation. (Palpate the calves and areas behind the knees for tenderness or pain.)

Preoperative EKG. Any patient with a history of heart disease or with signs and symptoms associated with heart disease undergoes a preoperative EKG. (In some hospitals, this is done routinely for all patients over age 35.) Immediately report any abnormal EKG findings.

GI status

Perioperative stress, anesthesia, and preoperative medications may cause nausea and vomiting. They also may be responsible for a postoperative decrease in intestinal muscle tone and motility, ranging from sluggish peristalsis to absence of motility in a segment of the small intestine (paralytic ileus). Because of this risk, you'll want to examine the patient's abdomen preoperatively for any of the following signs and symptoms of GI problems:
• Abdominal distention: Is the patient's abdomen taut and protruding? Firm on palpation?
Rationale: A tight, distended abdomen may point to hepatic, gastric, or intestinal problems.
• Bowel sounds: What is the character of the patient's bowel sounds (present, absent, diminished, or hyperactive)? Are sounds audible in all four quadrants of the abdomen?
Rationale: Absent, diminished, or hyperactive and loud bowel sounds may indicate a problem with GI motility and peristalsis. Report abnormal findings immediately.

Urinary-renal status. Urine retention may result from anticholinergic, antihistaminic, or sedative medications used during the perioperative period or from overdistention of the bladder. If the patient is scheduled for a prolonged procedure or one in which distention of the bladder might interfere with surgery, he may be catheterized before the procedure. The patient also may need catheterization if his urine output requires hourly monitoring.

If the patient requires catheterization preoperatively, be sure to assess for signs and symptoms of urinary tract infections and to monitor urine output. Note the following:
• Is the preoperative urinalysis normal? Report any abnormal findings to the doctor immediately.
Rationale: Although the patient may be asymptomatic, urinalysis often reveals infections or other potentially serious problems.

• Does the patient often feel the urge to urinate? Does he experience pain or bleeding on urination?
Rationale: These signs and symptoms indicate bladder infection and should be reported to the doctor.
• Has the patient ever experienced bladder or kidney problems? If so, when was the last episode? Is he currently experiencing back pain in the area of the kidneys? Are the kidneys tender to palpation or blunt percussion?
Rationale: A patient with chronic renal problems may have impaired renal function. This requires further examination by a doctor, who may order special tests to ensure the patient's renal function is sufficient to withstand the added stress of surgery.
• Does the male patient have urgency, frequency, nocturia (more than two times per night), diminished urine stream, or incomplete bladder emptying?
Rationale: A patient with prostatic hypertrophy is at increased risk for postoperative urine retention and may require further evaluation and intervention before surgery.

2 General Perioperative Care

This section includes general information on patient care during the entire perioperative period. For more specific information on the perioperative care of patients undergoing various types of surgery, see Section 5.

☐ Preoperative period

Regardless of the type of surgery, you'll want to safeguard your patient's well-being and prevent or minimize complications. To do so, you can incorporate the following information into your care plans.

Patient teaching

Throughout your other rotations, patient teaching may not have been an extensive part of your nursing responsibility. However, in surgery, patient teaching is considered a top priority. This is because the most common causes of surgical complications and death arise from problems that often could have been prevented.

Studies indicate that patients who receive preoperative teaching have less difficulty with anesthesia and a less complicated recovery. Once you learn the rationale behind preoperative teaching, you can not only teach your patient how to avoid postoperative complications but also motivate him to cooperate with the prescribed postoperative regimen.

Follow these general guidelines to ensure that your patient understands the sequence of events involving his surgery and that he can participate actively in making his preoperative period safe and uncomplicated.

Preventing respiratory complications

The most common causes of death or complications in patients who receive anesthesia include atelectasis, pneumonia, acute respiratory failure, and pulmonary emboli. You can teach your patient certain techniques to prevent these complications, such as techniques to keep the lungs' alveoli open, to expel excess secretions from the lungs, and to prevent stasis and clotting of blood in the extremities.

Begin by explaining that anesthesia causes the lungs to produce excess secretions which, if not expelled, could lead to serious complications. During anesthesia, respirations are shallow and the lungs are not well aerated. Secretions pool in the small outer airways, causing them to clog.

Explain to the patient that, even though he may not feel chest congestion or the urge to cough or deep-breathe, he will need to perform respiratory exercises to loosen the secretions deep in the bases of his lungs. These exercises include breathing techniques to help expand and aerate his lungs and coughing exercises to help expel mucus. Also explain that you'll be teaching him leg exercises to stimulate circulation and prevent blood clotting from immobility.

Deep-breathing exercises. Teach the patient the following deep-breathing exercises:

Flow-incentive spirometry (voluntary sustained maximal inspiration). Of the two types of incentive spirometers (flow and volume), the flow-incentive spirometer is the type most commonly used. It helps the patient take slow, deep breaths, thereby creating high transpulmonary pressures to keep the alveoli open and inflated.

Patient guidelines for use are as follows:
• Hold the spirometer upright or set it on a flat surface (tilting it will decrease the amount of inspiratory effort required to lift the device's balls).
• Inhale slowly through the mouthpiece, keeping the balls raised for the count of three.
• Exhale.
• Be sure to cough after each session to expel secretions. (The sole purpose of the spirometer is to move air in and out of the alveoli to mobilize secretions.)
• Take at least five normal breaths between each exercise, and repeat the exercise 10 times during each waking hour.
• Avoid using the spirometer after meals because nausea may result.

Voluntary deep breathing. Deep breathing hyperventilates the alveoli by keeping them open and inflated during the period of sustained inspiration. It also mobilizes secretions trapped in the smaller airways.

Patient guidelines for deep breathing are as follows:
• Lie in semi-Fowler's position with a pillow beneath your head.
• With your hands placed on each side of your chest, inhale slowly, holding your breath to a count of three. (Your hands should feel the expansion of your rib cage.)
• Exhale slowly and completely.
• Repeat the exercise three times every hour during the first postoperative day, then every hour until resuming your usual activity level.

Coughing exercises. Alveoli become inflated and aerated only during the inspiratory, or deep-breathing, phase of the respiratory exercise. Coughing, a postoperative expiratory maneuver, mobilizes lung secretions so that they can be expelled if the lungs are congested. Usually contraindicated in patients who have undergone eye or ear surgery, neurosurgery, or large abdominal hernia repair, coughing also may be restricted in other surgeries at the doctor's discretion.

If your patient is expected to cough postoperatively, explain the need for coughing despite its discomfort and not feeling the need to do so. Also, tell him that pain medications can be given before coughing exercises and that his abdomen can be splinted with a pillow to decrease the pain (if he underwent abdominal, thoracic, or pelvic surgery).

Instruct the patient to do the following:
• Sit on the side of the bed with your feet supported, if you can maintain this position. If not, lie in semi-Fowler's position.
• Place a pillow over your abdomen, and clasp your hands around the front of it.
• Inhale slowly and deeply through the nose, hold for a count of three, then exhale slowly. Do this three times.
• Inhale and hold your breath for a count of three.
• Cough three times to exhale.
• Inhale slowly, then cough immediately two more times.
• Repeat the exercise twice in succession, as tolerated.
• Follow coughing with deep breathing to reexpand the alveoli.

Exercises to prevent problems from immobility. After surgery, patients naturally tend to remain as still as possible to prevent pain from movement. However, prolonged inactivity during the postoperative period may lead to such complications as pulmonary embolus, lung congestion, paralytic ileus, decubitus ulcers, or contractures.

Your job is to educate and motivate the patient by making sure he understands the reasons for mobility exercises and by teaching him the following:

Sitting. Assist the patient to a sitting position, if this is not contraindicated. Sitting at least once every 4 hours will improve ventilation, prevent dependent edema of the back and sacrum, and improve circulation. Teach the patient to raise himself to a sitting position by turning on his side with his body in alignment, placing his palms on the mattress, and pushing himself up while swinging his feet around to a sitting position.

Turning. If the patient cannot sit upright, teach him to turn from side to side at least every 2 hours using the bed's raised side rails and his legs (if he is able to do so).

Leg exercises. Explain to the patient that not moving his legs after surgery can cause blood pooling, clotting, and joint stiffness.

Teach him the following exercises (if not contraindicated) to improve circulation and keep joints flexible:

Set 1
• Begin in semi-Fowler's position with your hips in alignment.
• Bring the knee of one leg up toward your chest with the calf parallel to the bed and the foot flexed.
• Extend the leg and lower it to the bed.
• Repeat five times with each leg.
Set 2
• Point the toes of both feet toward the head of the bed, then relax your feet.
• Point the toes toward the foot of the bed, then relax your feet.
• Repeat five times in each direction each hour while in bed.
Set 3
• Make a circular motion with your ankles in one direction; then repeat the motion in the opposite direction.
• Repeat five times each hour while in bed.
Set 4
• Place your feet approximately 1½" (3.8 cm) apart with the heels remaining on the mattress.
• Point your toes toward each other, then outward, rotating your hip joint.
• Repeat five times each hour while in bed.

Activity progression

The return of preoperative mobility usually begins the first post-operative day; however, be sure to check with your instructor and review doctor's orders for each individual patient. Depending on the type of surgery the patient is undergoing, explain that his activity may progress postoperatively as follows:

Leg dangling. If not contraindicated by the type of surgery or the patient's postoperative condition, the patient may be allowed to sit on the side of the bed and dangle his legs for 5 to 10 minutes. Be sure to stay with the patient at this time in case he becomes dizzy or syncopal.

To prevent edema and stasis in the legs, lower the bed and provide a footstool for the patient to rest his legs. If the patient complains of light-headedness, return him to a recumbent position and take his blood pressure. Report any continued complaints of syncope to your instructor or the charge nurse.

Out-of-bed orders. Leg dangling usually is followed by out-of-bed orders that may include assisted walks to the bathroom. As the patient progresses, he may be permitted to sit upright in a chair and to ambulate as tolerated. *Note:* When in doubt about the patient's activity level, always check the doctor's orders. Do not depend on the patient to know what he is allowed to do.

Preoperative patient preparation

The preoperative period is one of great anxiety for most patients, regardless of the type of surgery scheduled. For the nurse, this is a period involving various routines associated with preparing the patient for the operative procedure. The following information will help to familiarize you with the usual routines and to prepare a general care plan.

General preparation guidelines

Adequate patient preparation is a prerequisite for any surgical procedure. Routine preoperative procedures include the following:

The operative permit. A surgeon cannot operate on a patient without the patient's permission. The purpose of obtaining an operative permit is twofold: to protect the patient from unwanted surgery and to protect the surgeon from the liability of performing a surgical procedure without the patient's consent.

Before signing the permission form, the patient should understand what surgery is to be performed, when it is to be done, what complications and risks are associated with the procedure, and how body parts will be disposed of, if applicable. The surgeon is responsible for explaining the procedure to the patient and obtaining his permission. The nurse is responsible for evaluating the patient's understanding of the procedure.

At times, the surgeon may ask you to witness the signing of the operative permit. If this should occur, you may wish to have your instructor present. Ask the patient if he understands what the surgeon has explained and have him discuss what has been said. If the patient apparently understands and agrees to the procedure, you may sign your name after the patient's signature. If he does not seem to understand, notify your instructor and the patient's doctor. Remember, if you have any concern about the patient's comprehension, be sure to question him before signing the consent form. (*Note:* A surgical consent form should be signed *before,* not after, the administration of preoperative medications.)

A patient must sign his own consent. If he cannot do so for reasons of unconsciousness or mental incompetence or because he is a minor, a family member or legal guardian must sign. A surgeon can perform a lifesaving procedure without consent, but he must show proof that he attempted to contact the family by phone (witnessed call) or telegram.

The signed operative permit, usually obtained the day or night before surgery, is a permanent part of the patient's chart. However, it is legal only for a certain period after the witnessed signing. Some hospitals require additional consents for such surgeries as tubal ligations and vasectomies. Be sure to check your hospital's policy.

NPO status. The surgical patient is usually placed on NPO status—that is, he can receive nothing by mouth—beginning at midnight on the day of surgery. Make sure the patient's bed and intake and output sheets are tagged "NPO," and explain to the patient what this means. Be specific, and tell him he can have no food or fluids, including water.

If your patient is diabetic, check doctor's orders for how to handle the patient's fast. If the patient is scheduled to undergo regional or local anesthesia, he may be permitted to eat a light breakfast.

Preoperative shower. For most patients, a shower using an antimicrobial soap is ordered before surgery. Sometimes, the patient may be asked to cleanse the anticipated surgical site for 5 minutes, scrubbing in a circular motion.

Sleeping medication. Explain to the patient that medication is necessary to ensure a good night's rest. Mention that he will receive another injection or oral medication (or both) immediately before surgery to relax and prepare him for anesthesia.

Family teaching and support. Tell the patient's family what time they must arrive if they wish to visit the patient before surgery. Show them the surgical waiting area and tell them who to contact during the surgery if they have questions. Instruct them to inform the secretary or volunteer before leaving the surgical waiting area so they can be contacted if necessary. Encourage them to ask questions and to share their concerns.

Special preparations. The patient may require bowel, gastric, vaginal, or urinary preparation as well as any other special preparatory measures ordered by the doctor. Common preparations are listed below:

Bowel preparation. Bowel preparation (when ordered) depends on the type and location of the surgery. You can expect the patient undergoing colon or rectal surgery to receive laxatives, an enema, a low-residue or clear-liquid diet, or antibiotics (or a combination of these). Check the routine policy on your unit and doctor's orders.

Note: When "enemas until clear" are ordered, the doctor should be notified after the third try if the order is unsuccessful. Remember, repeated enemas can cause electrolyte imbalances (especially fluid retention and potassium depletion). If not contraindicated, give the patient a glass of apple juice to drink between enemas to replace sodium and potassium losses.

Gastric precautions. The doctor may order gastric intubation for removing possible residual stomach contents or various other reasons. (For instructions on inserting and caring for a nasogastric tube, see Section 5.)

Vaginal preparation. The doctor may request that the female patient receive a medicated douche before undergoing gynecologic or urologic procedures. Follow routine standing orders on your unit for this procedure.

Urinary preparation. Preoperative medications and overdistention of the bladder can cause loss of bladder tone. To prevent postoperative urine retention, a urinary catheter may be ordered. If the surgery is a short procedure, the patient may need only to void before surgery.

The morning of surgery

On the morning of your patient's scheduled surgery, expect to perform the following procedures:

Morning blood work. Check the patient's morning preoperative blood work. Report any abnormal findings to the doctor immediately, if he is not already aware of them. In particular, report:
- hemoglobin level less than 10 g/dl
- hematocrit level less than 33%
- potassium level greater than 5.3 mEq/liter or less than 3.5 mEq/liter
- urinalysis results indicating positive glucose or pyuria
- any abnormal coagulation studies (prothrombin time, partial thromboplastin time, or platelet count).

Also check to see that the patient's blood has been typed and crossmatched, if ordered.

Patient's chart. Make sure that all laboratory results, consultations, and permits are included in the patient's chart.

Physical assessment. Perform a brief physical assessment as close as possible to the time of surgery. Be sure to record the following:
- vital signs
- neurologic status, including level of consciousness and orientation
- cardiovascular status
- pulses
- heart sounds
- respiratory status, including respiratory rate, rhythm, and depth and breath sounds
- renal and urinary status, including urine color and output (measure output according to catheter collection bag's graduated markings, or have the patient void), urinary catheter patency, and the condition of the bladder on palpation
- skin status, including skin color and the condition of the skin surrounding the surgical site.

Before releasing the patient to the operating room

Immediately before releasing the patient to the operating room for surgery, be sure to do the following:
- Ask the patient to perform a brief session of coughing and deep breathing to clear any secretions that have accumulated during the night.

• Check to see that the patient has a legible identification band. If not, obtain a new one.
• Prepare the patient's chart, making sure it includes the following:
  —operative permit
  —preoperative blood work results
  —doctor's history and physical examination records
  —surgeon's progress notes
  —intake and output record
  —up-to-date nurses' notes
  —highlighted special orders (concerning diabetes, allergies, or other special problems).
• Remove items that the patient might lose, that may interfere with the surgery, or that may prove harmful to the patient during surgery, including:
  —makeup
  —jewelry
  —hairpins
  —nail polish
  —artificial nails
  —dentures or partial plates
  —prostheses.
Note: Although some hospitals may allow a wedding ring or other special ring (such as a religious ring) to be taped to the patient's finger, it is best to remove all rings and give them to the patient's family or have them placed in the hospital safe. Overhydration, especially which may occur in major surgeries, can cause edema of the fingers. In such operations as cardiac bypass surgery, severe postoperative edema may occlude circulation distal to the ring.
• Document the administration of preoperative medication. Record the time you received the call from the operating room, the medication given, the dose and route, and the time the medication was administered. Explain to the patient that the injection will relax him and ease the induction of anesthesia. Make sure the bed side rails remain upright, and instruct the patient to stay in bed after receiving the injection or oral medication.

Nursing diagnoses
The following nursing diagnoses are associated with the preoperative period:
• Altered Nutrition: Less Than Adequate for Uncomplicated Surgical Recovery related to (state etiology)
• Anxiety related to altered body image or function
• Anxiety related to surgery or possible adverse surgical findings
• Fluid Volume Deficit: Less Than Adequate for Surgery related to (state etiology)

• Grieving related to anticipated loss of body function or body part
• Ineffective Family or Individual Coping (or both) related to surgery
• Knowledge Deficit related to the immediate preoperative and postoperative events
• Knowledge Deficit related to postoperative rehabilitation (if applicable)
• Knowledge Deficit related to potential postoperative pulmonary complications
• Knowledge Deficit related to the surgical procedure
• Knowledge Deficit related to techniques for clearing bronchial secretions
• Spiritual Distress related to conflicts between religious beliefs and prescribed treatments (such as blood transfusions).

☐ Operative period

Because most nursing students merely observe in the operating room (OR) and do not assist with procedures, this section does not include a detailed description of OR nursing. Discuss your specific role in the OR with your instructor and charge nurse before your patient's surgery. Also, be sure to obtain the surgeon's permission to observe the procedure, and adhere to his rules concerning the role of observers.

As an observer in the OR, you'll want to review strict aseptic technique and be familiar with gowning and gloving procedures. Also familiarize yourself with the surgery to be performed and review the various surgical techniques commonly used in the procedure. If implantable devices are part of the procedure, make sure you know their purpose.

As a general rule, remain out of the immediate operative field unless you're asked to view a procedure closely. However, feel free to ask questions of the nursing and OR staff about the OR environment, surgery, anesthesia, equipment, or other special procedures.

☐ Postoperative period

Perhaps at no other time does the nurse play such a vital role in patient care as when observing patients during the postoperative period. Known as the period of "eternal vigilance" during which lack of attention to even small details can result in major problems for the patient, the postoperative period is divided into two phases: immediate recovery and general postoperative. During these phases, the nurse works independently, routinely observing for signs or symptoms of possible complications.

Throughout the entire postanesthesia recovery period, you'll need to do the following:
• Perform neurologic checks (sensory and motor responses, level of consciousness) every 15 minutes (for information on the return of reflexes and level of consciousness, see the following page).
• Take and record vital sign measurements every 15 minutes.
• Assess the airway for patency, and suction as needed.
• Assess respiratory status.
• Assess the condition of surgical dressings.
• Monitor all I.V. lines and drainage tubes.
• Monitor urine output at least every half hour (in a catheterized patient).
• Determine the need for catheterization if the bladder is distended and the patient cannot void.

Immediate recovery period

As a nursing student, you may have the opportunity to assist in the recovery of an anesthetized surgical patient under the supervision of your instructor or a nurse specially trained in postoperative recovery. Before your patient arrives from the OR, check to see that all equipment necessary to recover the patient is at the bedside.

Depending on the surgery, you will need at least the following items:
• equipment to open, clear, or reestablish the airway
• oxygen source with a new bubble bottle and tubing
• suction device
• emesis basin and mouth wipes
• penlight to check pupillary response
• blankets for hypothermia
• anesthetic reversal agents
• medications for pain and laryngeal spasms or other respiratory problems
• equipment to take vital signs.

Check with the OR about any special needs the patient may have postoperatively, such as a ventilator or cardiac monitor. Know where to locate such emergency equipment as the crash cart and tracheostomy tray. While waiting for your patient's arrival, review your own unit's policy for preparing the patient cubicle and make sure that all items are in place.

When the patient arrives, observe him for the following events.

Return of reflexes and level of consciousness

When a patient recovers from anesthesia, reflexes return in the reverse order in which they disappeared: unconsciousness, response to stimuli, drowsiness, disorientation, and orientation.

Assess the patient every 5 to 15 minutes according to the criteria contained in the neurologic section of your unit's postanesthesia record. Most patients are oriented to person, place, and time within 1 hour after surgery, and the average stay in nonintensive care recovery is less than 2 hours.

The actual amount of contact you'll have with the patient will depend on the type of anesthetic he received. For example, a patient who received ketamine intraoperatively may hallucinate and will require a quiet recovery. During this time, avoid touching the patient or exciting him in any way.

Note: Take this opportunity to learn about various anesthetics and their recovery characteristics from your instructor or the postanesthesia care unit (PACU) nurse supervising your activities.

Airway obstruction, hemorrhage, and shock

To detect airway obstruction, hemorrhage, and shock—the primary immediate postoperative complications—assess the following areas promptly after the patient arrives in the PACU:

Airway

• With your hand placed over the patient's mouth or endotracheal (ET) tube, check the airway and feel for the amount of air exchange. Although breathing may be shallow, you should be able to feel it easily through the mouth or ET tube.

• Check bilaterally for rise and fall of the chest wall. However, don't assume that because the patient's chest is moving, he is breathing. Feeling for air through the nose and mouth is the only way to be sure. Bilateral chest wall expansion is a backup observation that reveals depth and equality of muscle excursion.

• Auscultate the lungs. You should hear breath sounds bilaterally. If breath sounds are absent on one side, the patient's ET tube may have become displaced and lodged in either mainstem bronchus.

• Note the presence or absence of a gag reflex by lightly touching the back of the oropharynx using the tip of a suction catheter. This will indicate whether the patient can clear his airway of mucous secretions.

Interventions (airway)

Problem: Unilateral breath sounds

This could indicate displacement of the ET tube or other major problems.

Action: Notify the supervising nurse or doctor. Repositioning of the ET tube may be required.

Problem: No air exchange

You cannot feel air by placing your hand over the patient's nose or mouth or over the ET tube. The chest may be still. Opening the airway reveals no respiration.

Action: Use an Ambu bag for a patient with an ET tube or attempt to ventilate the unintubated patient with an oral airway, Ambu bag, and mask. If this proves successful, the patient's apnea probably is caused by insufficient recovery from anesthesia or sedation. Notify the supervising nurse or doctor, as anesthetic reversal medications may be required. Remember, the nurse's primary responsibility is to help the patient breathe when he is unable to do so unaided. You may participate to the extent that you are permitted.

Problem: Obstruction

No air passes through the patient's mouth or nose or through the ET tube. The patient may be in distress, and attempts to ventilate him are unsuccessful.

Action: If the patient has no ET tube, open the airway by hyperextending the neck (if not contraindicated). Look, listen, and feel for breathing, then suction the oropharynx and check again for breathing. (Postoperative mucous secretions are the most common cause of obstruction.)

If you're unsuccessful in dislodging the obstruction, turn the patient on his side and follow basic life-support guidelines for obstruction until help arrives. Usually, the anesthesiologist will be called to examine the oropharynx and larynx with a laryngoscope to locate the problem. Laryngeal stridor (grunting and laboring on inspiration or expiration, or both) and, subsequently, laryngeal edema occasionally develop after intubation, causing obstruction. Immediately notify the doctor, who may order medications to relieve the problem.

Depending on the severity of the problem, reintubation may be necessary. If an oral airway is in place, check its position and suction the patient's oropharynx; then check respirations. When caring for a patient with an ET tube, suction the tube and attempt to ventilate with an Ambu bag. Notify the doctor if these measures do not restore breathing immediately.

Problem: Shallow breathing

Action: Check the patient's arterial blood gas (ABG) levels, if available, for indications of hypoventilation (decreased PaO_2 and increased $PaCO_2$). If ABG levels are unavailable, assess for cyanosis, especially around the mucous membranes. Notify the supervising nurse or doctor if the patient's condition appears to be deteriorating.

Problem: No gag reflex

Action: Turn the patient often from side to side, if permitted, to prevent pooling of secretions in the throat. Make sure the patient

RECOGNIZING THE STAGES OF SHOCK

Because shock is a dynamic process, your patient's stability is difficult to maintain; he may improve or deteriorate rapidly as the process reverses or progresses. Recognizing the signs and symptoms of each stage of shock will help you classify your patient's condition according to its severity so you can intervene appropriately.

Early or compensatory stage

- Restlessness, irritability, apprehension
- Slightly increased heart rate
- Normal blood pressure, or slightly elevated systolic pressure or slightly decreased diastolic pressure
- Mild orthostatic blood pressure changes (15 to 25 mm Hg)
- Normal or slightly decreased urine output
- Pale and cool skin in hypovolemic shock; warm and flushed skin in septic, anaphylactic, and neurogenic shock
- Slightly increased respiratory rate
- Slightly decreased body temperature (except fever in septic shock)

Intermediate or progressive stage

- Listlessness, apathy, confusion, slowed speech
- Tachycardia
- Weak and thready pulse
- Decreased blood pressure
- Narrowed pulse pressure (except widened in septic shock)
- Moderate to severe orthostatic blood pressure changes (25 to 50 mm Hg)
- Oliguria
- Cold, clammy skin
- Tachypnea
- Decreased body temperature

Late or decompensatory stage

- Confusion and incoherent, slurred speech, possibly unconscious
- Depressed or absent reflexes
- Slow-to-react, dilated pupils
- Slowed, irregular, thready pulse
- Decreased blood pressure with diastolic pressure reaching zero
- Oliguria or anuria
- Cold, clammy, cyanotic skin
- Slow, shallow, irregular respirations
- Severely decreased body temperature

Death

has an airway in place, and suction secretions as needed. Remember, the nurse is responsible for keeping the patient's airway clear until he can do so himself.

Hemorrhage and shock

A surgical patient in hypovolemic shock displays certain signs and symptoms usually related to hemorrhage or dehydration (although dehydration is unlikely during the immediate recovery phase). Shock occurs in three stages: early, intermediate, and late (see *Recognizing the stages of shock*).

If you suspect hypovolemic shock, perform the following assessment:
- Check the patient's level of consciousness against the last recorded report. (In shock, level of consciousness declines.)
- Check the patient's systemic blood pressure (should be greater than 90/60 or within 20 mm Hg of the last recorded blood pressure).
- Check for flat neck veins (usually present in hypovolemic shock).
- Check the patient's pulse rate. (In shock, the pulse rate increases as the blood pressure declines.)
- Monitor respirations. (Shock usually is marked by tachypnea.)
- Check the surgical dressing or wound site for obvious, excessive bleeding. (With serious hemorrhage, bleeding is usually copious and bright red, or swelling is apparent around the operative site. Internal abdominal bleeding usually is more difficult to detect.)
- Check the patient's urine output. (Shock causes oliguria.)

Interventions (hemorrhage and shock)
Problem: Hypovolemic shock
Blood pressure is less than 90/60 or drops significantly (20 mm Hg) from the last recorded intraoperative blood pressure measurement. (*Note:* Trends are more important than individual blood pressure measurements.) Look for a decreasing blood pressure with an increasing pulse rate. Skin pallor, cyanosis, or mottling and poor capillary refill time may also point to shock.
Action: Ensure airway patency and administer oxygen. Check the I.V. line for patency and administer fluids rapidly until you obtain a stable blood pressure or the doctor arrives. Place the patient in shock (straight Trendenlenburg) position, continually monitoring his blood pressure and level of consciousness. Then place the patient on a cardiac monitor. Monitor urine output and insert an indwelling (Foley) catheter if one isn't in place.

Problem: Visible wound hemorrhage resulting in shock
Action: Remove the dressing and identify the hemorrhage site. Using multiple surgical pads, place pressure on the area until the doctor arrives.

Septic shock. Septic shock, unlike hypovolemic shock (which causes decreased blood volume), results in the uneven distribution of blood throughout the circulatory system. This in turn leads to decreased peripheral resistance and the tendency for blood to pool in the capillaries. Causative organisms include viruses, fungi, and bacteria; however, after surgery, gram-negative sepsis occurs most commonly.

The following patients are at increased risk for developing sepsis after surgery and should be monitored closely: patients over age 65, patients with diabetes, and patients undergoing urologic or genitourinary procedures. Patients with debilitating diseases or indwelling catheters, such as central venous lines, also should be monitored closely for signs of septic shock.

Septic shock progresses through two phases: warm shock and cold shock. The earlier the disorder is detected, the greater the chance of patient survival. Signs and symptoms are as follows:

Warm shock
• Skin: warm, flushed
• Cardiac: tachycardia, full bounding pulse
• Respiratory: tachypnea, hyperventilation
• Central nervous system: restlessness and confusion
• Blood pressure: normal to decreased

Cold shock
• Skin: cool to cold and clammy
• Cardiac: tachycardia with thready pulse
• Respiratory: respiratory failure, pulmonary congestion
• Central nervous system: progressively declining level of consciousness
• Blood pressure: severely decreased (80/60 mm Hg).

If your patient appears to be in septic shock, notify your instructor or supervising nurse, who will help you take the following measures:
• Ensure airway patency, administer oxygen by cannula or mask, and monitor ABG levels.
• Make sure the patient is properly intubated if respiratory failure occurs (this will be done by trained personnel), and ventilate as necessary.
• Make sure the patient has a patent large-bore I.V. line in place; administer Ringer's lactate or normal saline solution at the ordered rate.
• Assist with obtaining the necessary materials for blood cultures.
• Culture any possible sites of existing infection, such as indwelling catheters and wounds.
• Monitor the patient if he has a central venous line or pulmonary artery catheter in place.
• Continuously monitor the patient's arterial pressure.
• Place the patient on a cardiac monitor and observe for dysrhythmias.
• Administer antibiotics, as ordered.

Postanesthesia recovery period

Each PACU has its own forms for admission and discharge criteria as well as flowcharts for continuing evaluation. Be sure to familiarize yourself with these forms and charts by visiting the unit before you begin your rotation.

The following criteria are indicated for patient discharge from the PACU to an area of nonspecialized care:

• The patient's gag reflex returns, and he can clear his own airway.

• The patient can turn himself on his side. (This mobility guards against aspiration of secretions or vomitus.)

• The patient has control of respiratory function as evidenced by adequate aeration and ventilation, normal respirations, and minimal secretions.

• The patient's systemic blood pressure is stable.

• The patient rouses easily, indicating that he is not oversedated. (The patient's orientation should be as recorded preoperatively, and his level of consciousness should meet your individual unit's criteria.)

• Dressings are intact, reinforced, or redressed so that no wound drainage penetrates through the dressing.

• All tubes and drains are patent.

• For patients with regional anesthesia, motor function and proprioception return.

If you're asked to report your patient's condition to a receiving nurse, you'll want to include the following information:

• type of surgery
• estimated blood loss
• type of anesthesia and any necessary special precautions
• any unusual occurrences
• a review of doctor's orders
• the patient's current level of consciousness
• any analgesics administered in the PACU
• the patient's vital signs, including respiratory status
• presence of any dressings or drains
• presence of any I.V. lines, as well as the type of I.V. solution and rate of administration
• intake and output records, including any recent voidings
• any special equipment, such as special beds, flotation mattresses, or foam pads, that may be required.

Nursing diagnoses

Nursing diagnoses associated with the postanesthesia recovery period include the following:

• Altered Cardiac Output, Decreased: Declining Physiologic Responses and Decreased Level of Consciousness related to hypovolemia from hemorrhagic shock

• Altered Comfort related to incisional pain

• Fluid Volume Deficit related to dehydration

• Fluid Volume Excess related to overhydration during surgery

• Impaired Gas Exchange related to decreased lung aeration secondary to immobility and anesthesia

• Impaired Gas Exchange related to hypoventilation secondary to accumulation of mucous secretions in the airways

• Ineffective Airway Clearance related to absence of gag reflex secondary to sedation.

General postoperative period

When the patient is discharged from the recovery room, you may be asked to readmit him to the general surgical unit. After you receive his report from the PACU nurse, introduce yourself to the patient and explain that, because the move from recovery to the general unit sometimes causes changes in a patient's condition, you may need to reassess him.

After admission to the general unit, you will need to perform neurologic checks and monitor vital signs every 15 minutes for at least the first hour. (Afterward, monitor vital signs every 30 minutes for 1 hour, followed by once every hour for 4 hours, then once every 4 hours for 24 hours.) You also will need to perform a complete baseline physical assessment. Focus your observations and interventions on the following common postoperative complications.

Atelectasis

The incomplete expansion of the lung or any portion of the lung, atelectasis occurs as a result of the plugging and eventual collapse of alveoli by mucous secretions in the terminal bronchi and bronchioles. These secretions may result from anesthesia or the presence of a preoperative respiratory disorder. Postoperatively, the patient may be susceptible to atelectasis because of pooling of secretions from depressed respiration, anesthesia, analgesia, or ineffective coughing resulting in the retention of secretions.

Check for atelectasis by auscultating the patient's chest for areas of diminished breath sounds and palpating the thorax for areas of decreased vocal fremitus. Interventions include the following:
• Teach the patient preoperatively how to clear his secretions and improve aeration (see "Preoperative period" in this section). Ensure that he follows this routine.
• Instruct the patient to turn, cough, and deep-breathe at least three times each hour.
• Encourage increased fluid intake (if not contraindicated) to liquefy secretions.
• Increase the patient's activity level, as tolerated and as ordered.
• Instruct the patient to perform incentive spirometry, if ordered.
• Monitor the effects of any medications administered by a respiratory therapist, such as mucolytics to further liquefy secretions and help the patient cough and expectorate effectively.

Pneumonia

An inflammatory response caused by a viral or bacterial infection, pneumonia results in inadequate gas exchange in all or any part of the lung. Postoperative pneumonia—most commonly caused by gram-negative bacteria—usually develops within a few days after surgery but may develop within hours after surgery in susceptible patients. A patient with pneumonia usually develops dyspnea and tachypnea and may complain of pleuritic chest pain, especially in the lung bases. In severe cases, fever (greater than 101° F. [38.3° C.]), chills, and hemoptysis may occur.

If you suspect your patient may have pneumonia, percuss his chest for dullness and auscultate for fine crackles and decreased breath sounds. Evaluate ABG levels, if available. Report your findings to the doctor along with any of the other signs mentioned above.

Nursing interventions include:
• maintaining adequate hydration
• using techniques to clear bronchial secretions (including tracheal suctioning and deep breathing)
• preventing immobility
• administering pain medications (Prescribed pain medications help the patient comply with therapy.)
• administering antibiotics (the treatment of choice for bacterial pneumonia), as ordered
• instructing patients at risk for developing pneumonia in pulmonary hygiene and reporting the following significant signs and symptoms: flulike symptoms, fever, productive cough, chest pain, shortness of breath, and painful respirations.

Aspiration

A medical emergency, aspiration involves the inhalation of gastric contents, food, liquids, or other foreign material into the tracheobronchial tree. Postoperatively, this usually results from regurgitation of stomach contents in a heavily sedated patient or a patient with an absent gag reflex. Aspiration of large quantities of stomach contents (associated with a mortality above 50%) results in chemical irritation from the extreme acidity of the contents. Postanesthesia aspiration may not be noticeable because of the sedated patient's inability to cough or to protect his airway.

Regurgitation, unlike vomiting, is a passive process indicated by gurgling in the throat and signs of airway obstruction. If you notice your patient is regurgitating, take the following measures to ensure his safety and avoid or decrease the risk of aspiration:
• Turn the head to one side and suction the mouth and oropharynx.
• Take necessary steps to clear the airway. If the patient regurgitates a large volume of vomitus, suction the contents with the blunt end of the suction tubing or a large Yankauer suction tip.
• Place the head in a dependent position, if possible.
• Notify the doctor immediately.

Medical treatment involves chest X-ray, possible intubation, ABG measurements, and placement of a nasogastric (NG) tube for gastric decompression.

Note: Massive aspiration usually does not occur in patients who receive nothing by mouth (NPO status) several hours before surgery. It occurs more often in patients who have undergone emergency surgery and in those who experience GI hemorrhage.

Hypovolemic and septic shock

See "Immediate recovery period" in this section for details.

Pulmonary embolism

In pulmonary embolism, a complete or partial obstruction develops in the pulmonary artery or in a branching artery inside the lung. It usually is caused by a blood clot that forms elsewhere in the body, such as the legs or pelvis, and travels to the heart. The heart's pumping action breaks the clot into smaller pieces that are released and follow the path of blood flow.

The size of the released clot fragments determines the severity of the problem. Large fragments may lodge in the pulmonary artery and completely obstruct blood flow to the lungs. If not surgically removed, death will result within minutes. Smaller-sized fragments may pass through the pulmonary artery and wedge in smaller vessels within the lung, creating an area of alveolar nonperfusion. If the clot does not dissolve in time to reestablish blood flow to the dying tissue, infarction of this area may result.

In moderate pulmonary embolism, the patient usually complains of severe substernal chest pain, tachypnea, and shortness of breath. He usually is diaphoretic, tachycardic, and extremely anxious, often sits upright, and exhibits signs of panic as he tries to breathe despite coughing and wheezing (often producing pink or blood-tinged sputum). The episode may be accompanied by fever, hemoptysis, pleural effusion, and a pleural friction rub. ABG levels may show hypocapnia (a low $PaCO_2$), hypoxemia (a low PaO_2), and respiratory alkalosis (pH greater than 7.45).

In massive pulmonary embolism, the patient exhibits signs and symptoms of circulatory shock caused by lack of forward blood flow through the heart. Findings usually include hypotension, diaphoresis, oliguria, dyspnea, tachycardia, and a rapidly deteriorating level of consciousness.

Both moderate and massive pulmonary emboli are considered medical emergencies. If you observe the sudden onset of any of the above signs and symptoms, notify the doctor immediately or call a code.

Diagnosis is based on ventilation-perfusion scans and pulmonary angiography, currently considered the most definitive tests for diagnosing pulmonary embolism. Ultrasonography may be the most reliable noninvasive test.

Once the diagnosis has been made, treatment—which is medical and collaborative—aims to prevent further embolization. Because most clots dissolve spontaneously, anticoagulation therapy with heparin is the immediate treatment to prevent further clot formation. The patient is then maintained on bed rest for a designated period. Hypotension, resulting from decreased cardiac output, usually is treated with dopamine or isoproterenol. Oxygen is administered continuously, usually by ventilation mask. Because pain and anxiety exacerbate the patient's condition, pain medications usually are ordered, as needed.

Patients at risk for pulmonary embolism include those undergoing pelvic or hip surgery, those who are chronically ill, and those with peripheral vascular disease. Such patients need special instructions on leg exercises, the necessity for antiembolism stockings, and the need to elevate the legs.

Fluid and electrolyte imbalances

Fluid and electrolyte imbalances are interdependent and a common postoperative complication. Usually, you'll need to monitor electrolyte levels daily after most inpatient surgeries. Review the patient's morning blood work (chemistry profile) each day to check for abnormal sodium, chloride, or potassium levels. Notify the doctor of any abnormal results.

Urine retention

A postoperative patient is retaining urine if he has normal kidney function and does not void within 10 hours after surgery (depending on his estimated blood loss and fluid replacement). The cause of retention varies with the type of surgery, type and route of anesthetic, and other factors, such as preoperative bladder function.

If your patient complains of discomfort or has not voided within 8 hours after surgery, palpate his bladder for signs of distention. A distended bladder differentiates urine retention from oliguria or anuria.

To help the patient void, try running a faucet so that he can hear it, pouring warm water over the perineum, stroking or applying ice to the inner thigh, and helping him assume a comfortable position for voiding. Notify the doctor if these measures prove unsuccessful. Medication or catheterization may be necessary.

Urinary tract infection

In postoperative patients, urinary tract infections usually result from the use of a Foley catheter and typically occur 3 to 5 days after surgery. Infection may be introduced into the bladder during the catheterization process by infiltration of bacteria inhabiting the urinary meatus or distal urethra. Bacteria also can enter the bladder by migrating up the outer or inner surface of the catheter after the catheter is in place or at any time the closed drainage system is disrupted, as with specimen collection.

If urine is allowed to collect in the drainage bag and tubing without proper drainage, bacterial growth will occur over time. For this reason, the drainage bag should always be kept in a dependent position, below the patient's bladder level. Keep this in mind when moving the patient. Always hook the drainage bag to the bottom of the stretcher or bed; never toss it on the bed, where it will be at the same level as a reclining patient.

Signs and symptoms of urinary tract infection in a catheterized patient include elevated temperature and foul-smelling or bloody urine. The patient also may complain of pelvic, flank, or back pain. In an uncatheterized patient, signs and symptoms include urinary frequency and urgency, burning or pain on urination, oliguria, and sometimes fever (99° to 101° F. [37.2° to 38.3° C.]). Report signs and symptoms to the doctor immediately.

Urinary tract infection usually is diagnosed by urine culture and treated with appropriate antibiotics. Collaborative nursing interventions include ensuring the patient receives adequate hydration by encouraging fluids and maintaining an aseptic bladder drainage system.

Paralytic ileus

A common postoperative complication, paralytic ileus refers to the absence of peristalsis in all or part of the bowel. Related disorders include adynamic ileus (uncoordinated peristalsis) and sluggish or slow peristalsis. Paralytic ileus (or a related disorder) usually results from disruption of autonomic control of the bowel by medications (such as anesthetics and anticholinergics), surgical manipulation of the bowel, electrolyte imbalances, or other surgery-related events. It usually resolves within 48 to 72 hours after surgery.

A patient with this condition may have slight abdominal distention and absent bowel sounds. (Because bowel sounds may be diminished and difficult to hear, be sure to auscultate the abdomen for 1 minute in each quadrant before confirming their absence.) He typically passes no flatus or feces. After 12 to 24 hours, his abdomen may become tight and distended, and vomiting may occur from gastric distention.

If the patient's bowel sounds haven't returned within 16 hours after surgery, alert the doctor, who will order that the patient be given nothing by mouth (NPO status) until bowel sounds return. Observe for mild cramps, return of bowel sounds, and passage of flatus. These signs and symptoms indicate the return of peristalsis.

If the patient becomes excessively uncomfortable, the doctor may order medication to increase intestinal motility. If the patient has nausea and vomiting, an NG or other long intestinal tube (Abbott or Cantor) may be inserted by the doctor to decompress the stomach or bowel.

Keep in mind that mobility aids the return of peristalsis. Encourage the patient to walk frequently, if not contraindicated. Because all NPO patients are at risk for dehydration, monitor the patient's I.V. intake and urine output and electrolyte studies, and report any significant imbalances.

Nursing diagnoses

Nursing diagnoses associated with the general postoperative period include the following:

• Activity Intolerance related to postoperative pain and fatigue
• Altered Cardiac Output, Decreased related to circulatory shock
• Altered Comfort: Pain related to surgical incision
• Altered Tissue Perfusion, Renal: Decreased Output related to postanesthesia complications
• Disturbance in Self-Concept related to change in body image resulting from surgery
• Fluid Volume Deficit related to insufficient fluid replacement during and after surgery
• Fluid Volume Excess related to overhydration during or after surgery
• Impaired Gas Exchange related to atelectasis and pneumonia
• Impaired Mobility related to surgical incision or postoperative complications
• Impaired Skin Integrity related to wound drainage or immobility
• Impaired Tissue Integrity, Wound: Necrosis related to infection and lack of sufficient blood supply to wound surface
• Ineffective Airway Clearance related to sedation and poor cough reflex
• Ineffective Breathing Pattern related to painful incision
• Infection related to contamination of surgical wound, urinary bladder, or lungs (specify)
• Knowledge Deficit related to clearing secretions and aerating the lungs
• Knowledge Deficit related to discharge instructions
• Knowledge Deficit related to medications
• Knowledge Deficit related to permitted activity level
• Knowledge Deficit related to preventing the formation of venous thrombi
• Knowledge Deficit related to rehabilitation procedures
• Self-Care Deficit (specify) related to pain of surgery or surgical complications
• Urine Retention related to effect of anesthetics, analgesics, or antiemetics on autonomic control of bladder.

3 Wound and Burn Care

General principles of wound care involve creating an external and internal environment conducive to wound healing. Dressing changes and aseptic technique ensure control of the wound's external environment to allow for optimal tissue growth. Adequate nutrition and antibiotics promote a healthy internal environment necessary for wound repair and prevention or control of infection. Even with complicated, infected surgical wounds, these basic principles remain the same.

☐ External wound care

Interventions related to the care of the wound's external environment depend on the type of healing process involved. The major types of wound repair include healing by primary union (first intention), secondary union (secondary intention), and tertiary union (third intention).

Primary union, the usual form of repair for an uncontaminated surgical incision, involves the direct approximation of two uninfected areas of tissue, which permits healing by proliferation of connective tissue elements.

Secondary union involves repair of an infected wound by allowing healing from the inside out without closure. Infected wounds differ from noninfected wounds by producing necrotic debris and exudate, loss of a greater amount of tissue in the healing process, formation of more granulation tissue, slower healing, and larger scars. Many of these factors can be controlled through external wound care interventions.

Tertiary union involves delayed primary closure of the wound. Examples include uninfected wounds that become infected and must be reopened and wounds considered too contaminated for initial closure, such as wounds from trauma, some orthopedic surgeries, and fasciotomies.

The optimal external environment for tertiary union wound repair, which is always handled aseptically, depends on the stage of the wound healing process. During the phase in which the wound is open, repair is handled much like a wound of secondary union. After surgical debridement and closure, repair is handled like a primary wound.

The uncontaminated (normal) wound

The original surgical dressing for a normal wound may be occlusive and usually is not removed the day of surgery unless the wound shows evidence of bleeding or excessive drainage or the patient complains frequently about incisional pain despite having received analgesic medication.

Before your first dressing change, familiarize yourself with the normal appearance of a primary surgical wound. Based on this data, you can evaluate your patient for abnormal signs and symptoms that may indicate complications. Normal observations are as follows:

• Skin color surrounding the wound should be normal. Local irritation in the form of redness surrounding the suture material at the skin line is considered a normal reaction. However, the area adjacent to the suture line itself should not be reddened or warm.

• The wound edges should be closely approximated with no large gaps in the suture line. Be sure to document in detail any deviation from normal.

• No excessive pressure on the suture line, as evidenced by pulling or tearing of the skin at the suture insertion sites, should occur.

• Bleeding should be minimal after most surgical procedures by the end of the first postoperative day. Document moderate to excessive bleeding by the number of dressing changes needed to keep the dressing dry.

• The amount and type of drainage vary with the type of surgery. After most procedures, drainage should be serosanguineous and odorless.

• Vital signs should be normal, indicating probable absence of internal bleeding or complications, such as infection.

Care of the closed suture line

Although the surgeon may elect to perform the first dressing change, you, as a nurse, are responsible for investigating any suspected problem by aseptically removing as much of the dressing as necessary to see the wound. Be sure to change any dressing that has wet through to the outside immediately because wetness provides a route for invasive bacteria. To change the dressings on primary incisions, consult your instructor or the charge nurse and follow the guidelines listed below:

• Check the nurses' notes or doctor's progress notes for the positions of any wound drains.

• Assemble the following materials: nonsterile gloves, a plastic bag to dispose of old dressings, sterile normal saline solution, a sterile basin, antibacterial lotion or ointment or other prescribed antibacterial-antifungal agent, nonadhesive (Telfa or Adaptic) dressings, 4" × 4" gauze wipes, tracheostomy dressing pads to surround drains, abdominal dressing pads (ABDs or Surgipads), tape, and sterile gloves. (*Note:* If you have never performed this procedure before, you may want to include a sterile drape to create a sterile field on the patient's tray table. This way, you can open all sterile materials onto the field and move the table closer for easy access.)

• Protect bed linens with linen savers.

• Instruct the patient about the dressing procedure.

• Open all sterile materials onto the sterile field using aseptic technique. This includes the sterile basin, which you'll fill halfway with sterile normal saline solution, being careful not to contaminate the field. Squeeze out the antibacterial lotion or ointment onto the sterile field, making sure it does not soak through the sterile field.

• Put on the nonsterile gloves and prepare the plastic bag for disposal of the old dressing.

• Remove the old dressing by placing one hand lightly over the dressing to secure it and removing the tape by pulling toward the dressing.

• When all tape is loose, attempt to remove the dressing by lifting it from one corner. If the dressing appears to be adhering painfully to the wound, pour a small amount of sterile normal saline solution to the adhesion until the dressing comes off easily.

• Dispose of the dressing and nonsterile gloves in the plastic bag.

• Inspect the wound according to the criteria listed under "The uncontaminated (normal) wound," page 37. Remember any abnormal or suspicious areas to document in your record.

• Put on sterile gloves.

• Gently cleanse the suture line using the 4″ × 4″ gauze wipes soaked in normal saline solution. Starting at the top, wipe toward the bottom, using a different pad with each downward motion to gently remove any crusted areas. Dry the area with a separate gauze pad. Dispose of all pads in the plastic bag as you use them.

• Using your sterile gloved finger or the tip of a folded gauze pad, apply the antibacterial lotion or ointment (which had been dispensed earlier onto the sterile field) directly to the suture line. Apply from top to bottom; do not rub it into the skin.

• Apply a nonadhesive (Telfa or Adaptic) dressing over the suture line. Place gauze tracheostomy dressings around drain sites. Cover the area with dry 4″ × 4″ gauze followed by the outer surgical pad or gauze bandage.

• Measure and cut the desired amount of tape. After centering the tape over the wound dressing, apply gentle pressure, working outward bilaterally and making sure the tape adequately adheres to the skin surface. Most uninfected wounds do not require that the entire dressing or dressing border (occlusive dressings) be sealed with tape. Use just enough tape to keep the dressing securely in place.

• Document the quality and quantity of drainage and the appearance of wounds and drains.

Suture or staple removal

Suture removal may be requested by the doctor when he decides the wound has completed the healing process. Facial sutures usually are left in place for 3 days; most other sutures are ready for removal after 7 to 10 days.

To remove simple, interrupted sutures safely, use the following guidelines under the supervision of a nurse or your instructor:
• Obtain a suture removal kit, nonsterile gloves, and antiseptic solution to cleanse the wound.
• Ask if the patient has had sutures removed before. If not, explain that removal is painless but that he may experience slight discomfort if the sutures are tight or encrusted with dried blood.
• Protect bed linens with plastic linen savers.
• After putting on nonsterile gloves, cleanse the suture line with hydrogen peroxide on a sterile 4" × 4" gauze wipe or cotton-tipped applicator. (Hydrogen peroxide facilitates the removal of old blood and debris from the suture area.) Wipe the wound from top to bottom, soaking encrusted areas as you progress downward. Use a new sterile wipe or applicator with each downward motion until you are satisfied the wound is clean. (*Note:* The cleaner you can get the suture line, the easier the sutures can be removed. Don't be afraid to clean the wound vigorously, even if this is slightly uncomfortable for the patient. Keep in mind that the wound is healed and that suture removal will be more painful if you don't first remove the debris adhering to the sutures.)
• Using the forceps in your suture removal kit, grasp the top suture and pull it upward, away from the skin. (This may be difficult if sutures are tight or have been left in place too long. Do the best you can. Remember, this procedure will not reopen a healed wound.)
• Using the sterile scissors from your kit, clip the suture at the skin line on one side. Then, using the forceps, pull the suture out from under the skin on the opposite side. (*Note:* The principle of suture removal is to avoid pulling suture material previously outside the wound through the suture tract. If you clip the suture extremely close to the skin, you can avoid contaminating the internal suture tract, thereby preventing a possible infection.)
• Remove remaining sutures in the same manner as above.

Removing surgical staples involves the same cleansing technique used with suture removal. However, to remove the staples, you'll need a staple removal kit, which contains a special instrument that lifts the staple off the skin and bends it to release both

staple ends simultaneously. If you are unfamiliar with this procedure, read the directions on the kit and work under the supervision of your instructor or an experienced nurse.

Care of the open wound

Open wounds heal by secondary union, as tissue granulation
causes healing from the bottom of the wound toward the skin
surface. Each surgeon has his own preference for care of open
wounds. Although this can be particularly confusing at times,
you'll need to keep in mind the general principles of open
wound care to better understand why certain dressings are being
used and to create dressings specific to your patient's needs.

General principles of open wound care are as follows:
• Dry open wounds must be kept moist so that tissue regenera-
tion can occur, as cells cannot proliferate in a dry environment.
Sterile, damp 4″ × 4″ gauze wipes (usually soaked in normal
saline solution) placed against the open tissue will provide the
desired effect.
• Open wounds that are wet and draining produce exudate and
necrotic debris that must be removed to promote the formation
of healthy granulation tissue. Absorbent dressings are required to
control this excess drainage and to debride the wound (remove
dead tissue).
• Irrigation is used when necrotic tissue adheres to the wound
tissue or when topical antibiotic treatment is desired. Irrigation
also is used with sinus tracts, cavities, and penetrating wounds.
• Fistulas and continuously draining wounds may require drainage pouches, such as those used for ostomies. Skin surrounding
these wounds must be protected from prolonged contact with
wound drainage because this results in excoriation and skin
breakdown.

Managing the dry open wound

Your objective in managing the dry open wound is to provide a
moist environment that will encourage granulation and prevent
infection. Follow these guidelines:
• Assemble supplies for a primary dressing change (see *Dressing
materials for surgical wounds,* pages 42 and 43). Include extra
materials needed for a damp packing, depending on the size of
the wound, and an extra pair of sterile gloves. In damp-to-dry
dressings, 4″ × 4″ gauze wipes and individually packaged rolled
gauze (Kling or Kerlix) often are used. (*Note:* Antiseptic or antifungal medications, such as povidone-iodine and hexachlorophene, can cause tissue reactions when placed in direct contact
with open wounds if they are not rinsed after application. These
substances should not be used to pack a wound without the sur-

DRESSING MATERIALS FOR SURGICAL WOUNDS

Preparation	Commercial name	Method of use	Action	Comments
CLEANSING AGENTS				
Swabs	Cotton balls	Use cotton balls to apply solution	Remove debris by friction	May shed threads onto the wound
	Gauze	Use to apply solution and dry the wound	Removes debris by friction and absorbs moisture	May shed threads and catch on sutures
	Nonwoven gauze	Same as for gauze	Same as for gauze	Softer, less likely to shed
	Sponge sticks or swabs	Use to apply solution and dry the wound	Same as for gauze	Do not shed or catch; less malleable than gauze or cotton balls
DRESSINGS				
Gauze		Apply directly to the wound	Protects and absorbs exudate	Varies in thickness; several layers may be needed to prevent strike through; sticks when dry
Nonwoven gauze	Nugauze	Same as for gauze	Same as for gauze	Still adherent but more absorbent than cotton gauze; may have an internal absorbent layer
Nonstick pads	Melolite*, Release*, Selopor*, Telfa*	Same as for gauze	Same as for gauze	Less adherent than those above but still stick if allowed to dry out; synthetic pads
Foam dressing		Same as for gauze	Same as for gauze	Nonadherent surface
Wound contact layer	Adaptic*, Intersorb*, Jelonet*†, Nterface*	Same as for gauze	Protects surface epithelium from sticking to the dressing, which may be changed without removing this layer	Good for surface wounds with skin loss; reduces damage caused during dressing changes
Semi-occlusive or moisture vapor permeable	Bioclusive*, Ensure-it*, Opraflex*, Op-Site*, Tegaderm*, Thin Film*, UniFlex*	Same as for gauze	Protects wound; allows observation; supports the suture line	Useful for simple wounds, particularly in young children who need to be bathed; good for skin donor sites where they may be left until they drop off
Occlusive	DuoDerm*, Vigilon*	Same as for gauze	Protects wound; allows observation; supports the suture line	

DRESSING MATERIALS FOR SURGICAL WOUNDS *(continued)*

Preparation	Commercial name	Method of use	Action	Comments
Absorption pads	ABD Pad	Apply over the initial gauze or coated layer	Absorb exudate; layered pads contain extra absorbent materials	Made in set sizes; liable to come apart if cut to shape
Island dressings	AirStrip*, BandAid*, Coverlet O.R.*, Hypafix Post-OP*, Mepore*, Primapore*, Telfa-Plus*	Apply directly to wound	Absorbs and protects	May be used immediately postsurgery for small wounds without too much exudate, or later to replace a bulk dressing
TAPES				
Cloth	Elastoplast*, Zinc oxide	Use to attach dressings or as part of an island dressing to attach dressings	May cause allergy in sensitive patient	Used where support is required; strong for support
Hypoallergenic	Dermilite*, Micropore*, Selofix*	Use to attach dressings	Is hypoallergenic	General purpose tapes
	Hypafix*, Mefix*	Use to attach dressings; flexible	Is hypoallergenic	General purpose tapes
	Blenderm*	Use as water-repellent attachments	Is hypoallergenic	General purpose tapes
Waterproof	Elastoplast*, Plastic tape	Use where waterproof dressing is required; cover the dressing	Is waterproof	For dressings likely to be contaminated with body fluids

*Trademark
†To be used only as ordered

geon's consent. In the absence of orders, use sterile normal saline solution for the dressing change.)
• Wash your hands.
• Instruct the patient on the dressing procedure.
• Use linen savers to protect bedding.
• Use nonsterile gloves to remove the outer dressing. Then use the extra pair of sterile gloves to remove the inner packing from the previous dressing. Note the quality and quantity of drainage. Be careful not to leave any gauze wipes in the recesses of large wounds. Dispose of gloves and all soiled dressing materials in a plastic bag.
• Inspect the wound, looking for necrotic areas and accumulations of purulent material. Note any granulation (reddish-white

grainy material) at the bottom of the wound and any abnormal odors. The inside of the wound should be moist and pink. Soiled dressings should be moist, not dry, when removed.

• Prepare a sterile field on the patient's tray table. Open all sterile materials onto the disposable drape. Be sure to include a sterile basin to hold normal saline solution or the ordered medicated solution. Fill the basin with enough solution to prepare the dressing.

• Put on the second pair of sterile gloves and moisten the 4" × 4" gauze wipes (or whatever gauze packing the wound requires) in the basin. (*Note:* As a general rule, it is better to use continuous rolled gauze on wounds with small cavities and deep recesses; 4" × 4" gauze wipes can become lost in these tiny areas, but rolled gauze guarantees that all of the packing will be removed because it is continuous.) Squeeze the packing gauze to achieve the desired wetness. With dry open wounds, your aim is to wet the packing enough so that the packing remains damp through the next dressing change and does not adhere excessively to the wound.

• Pack the wound effectively, pressing the gauze gently to ensure it covers the entire interior surface. Continue to pack, using the same material, until the gauze is level with the skin surface.

• Cover the packing with gauze wipes and an outer surgical pad or gauze bandage.

• Tape the dressing in place using a nonocclusive outer dressing.

Managing the draining open wound

When managing a draining open wound, your objective is to remove exudate and necrotic debris with the dressing change. The type of dressing depends on the amount of drainage and how quickly it develops. The shape of the wound also plays a role in selecting the appropriate dressing. Follow the guidelines that appear most suited to the wound you are managing. Remember, large wounds may call for more than one approach; some areas may be dry while others are draining. Evaluate each section of the wound and dress it accordingly.

Strip packing

Strip packing is the dressing of choice after incision and drainage of an abcess or treatment of a puncture wound or any type of deep, narrow lesion that develops exudate and necrotic debris. Guidelines for strip packing are as follows:

• Administer pain medication 20 minutes before beginning the procedure.

• Assemble the following materials: a plastic bag, tape, povidone-iodine solution, sterile 4" × 4" gauze wipes, sterile gloves (two sets), sterile forceps, sterile scissors, and strip gauze (plain or iodoform, as ordered).

• Instruct the patient about the procedure.

• Use linen savers to protect bed linens.

• Using sterile gloves, gently peel away the soiled packing from the last dressing change to remove all of the gauze. (This may be uncomfortable for the patient, as the gauze is dry and packed deeply into the recesses of the wound.) Dispose of the gloves and gauze in a plastic bag. Note the quality and quantity of drainage.

• Open all materials aseptically and arrange them for use. Remember to lay caps of bottles upside down to protect sterility.

• Put on the second pair of sterile gloves. Use a sterile 4″ × 4″ gauze wipe moistened with povidone-iodine solution (if permitted) to wipe in a circular motion around the outer skin surface surrounding the wound. Repeat this process with a new gauze wipe.

• Using the sterile forceps, grasp the end of the strip gauze inside the bottle and estimate the amount needed; clip with sterile scissors. Hold one end of the gauze with your gloved hand and the other with the forceps. Begin packing with the forceps to the depth of the wound, folding the gauze over on itself as you progress outward and packing the wound until you reach the skin surface. Leave about a ½″ strip on the surface, and clip off the excess gauze.

• Cover the wound with 4″ × 4″ gauze wipes and secure with tape.

• Document your findings.

Wet-to-dry packing

Wet-to-dry dressings are handled in much the same manner as the damp-to-dry dressings used in dry open wounds. The objective here, however, is not to keep the wound moist (because the wound is draining) but to control infection and rid the wound of exudate and debris through the application of an absorbent dressing. Follow these guidelines for wet-to-dry packing:

• Assemble materials needed for a dry open wound dressing. Include povidone-iodine solution or whatever topical antibacterial treatment the surgeon orders.

• Protect bed linens with linen savers.

• Using nonsterile gloves, gently remove and dispose of the soiled dressing and gloves in a plastic bag. Note the quality and quantity of drainage.

• Inspect the wound. Excessive exudate and purulent drainage inside the wound indicates a need for more frequent dressing changes and drier packing. If these measures prove unsuccessful, contact your instructor and discuss the possibility of asking the surgeon about the use of irrigation or chemical debridement.

• Using sterile gloves, pack the wound level with the skin surface using a continuous roll gauze (Kling) or fine-mesh gauze moistened with povidone-iodine solution or the topical treatment ordered.

• Cover the wound with 4″ × 4″ gauze moistened with the same solution used to pack the wound, followed by dry 4″ × 4″ gauze, a Surgipad, and tape. If the wound tends to leak around the dressing, protect the skin with benzoin, zinc oxide, or another commercially available protectant and completely seal the edges of the dressing with waterproof tape.
• Document your findings.

Irrigation and chemical debridement

Wounds that produce necrotic debris inadequately removed by wet-to-dry dressings require irrigation, chemical debridement, or a combination of both methods.

With irrigation, the irrigating solution may be normal saline solution, a mixture of normal saline solution and hydrogen peroxide, or one of many variations of antiseptic and antifungal solutions. Follow doctor's orders for which irrigant to use; however, if no irrigating solution is specified, use normal saline solution.

The approach to irrigation also varies. The solution may be dispensed from a bulb syringe, a 50-ml piston syringe with an irrigation tip, a piston syringe with a sterile rubber catheter attached (to access the deep regions of the wound), or an I.V. bag of normal saline solution with an administration set and a large Teflon I.V. catheter attached (pressure is applied to the bag, and solution is released as a forceful stream through the I.V. catheter). Other devices include pressurized irrigators that dispense solution in intermittent bursts.

Keep in mind that, whichever administration method is used, the dispensing equipment and solution should be sterile. Your choice of method depends on equipment availability, doctor's orders, and the force needed to dislodge the debris. The choices given above begin with the most gentle method (bulb syringe) and end with the most forceful (jet action).

Chemical debridement is accomplished through the use of debriding ointment such as fibrinolysin and desoxyribonuclease (Elase). This ointment helps lift away dead tissue and promote healing from deep inside the wound. Chemically debrided wounds require irrigation with each dressing change to remove the previous ointment and adhering debris.

Use the following guidelines for irrigation and chemical debridement:
• Assemble materials necessary for a wet-to-dry dressing change. Decide on the method of irrigation, and gather the necessary materials, irrigant, and ointment. Cover the bed under the dressing with waterproof linen protectors. For some wounds, an emesis basin can be used to collect the irrigant that drains from the

wound. With other wounds, use towels and layers of linen savers to contain the drainage.
• Instruct the patient about the procedure.
• Using aseptic technique, open and arrange the dressing materials to be used for easy access.
• Using nonsterile gloves, remove and dispose of the soiled dressing, then the gloves, in a plastic bag. Note the quality and quantity of any drainage.
• Inspect the wound, looking for areas where necrotic debris (grayish-black pieces of tissue) has adhered to the wound. Vigorously irrigate these areas and attempt to remove the dead tissue. You may need to use a 4″ × 4″ gauze wipe simultaneously to cleanse the area with the flowing solution. Also look for healthy granulation tissue (pinkish-white and grainy). Gently irrigate over these areas to preserve the new growth.
• If you are irrigating an abdominal wound, place the patient in semi-Fowler's or a side-lying position. If you are irrigating an arm or leg or a wound elsewhere on the body, try to position the patient according to a superior-inferior gradient, with one part of the wound dependent. This will facilitate drainage.
• Fill the syringe or dispenser to be used with solution. Irrigate with a steady stream from the higher portion of the wound toward the lower portion of the wound, attempting to rinse away necrotic areas and heavy exudate. Be sure to irrigate inside the wound. Do not allow the solution to flow over the patient's skin, then into the wound.
• Dry the wound with 4″ × 4″ gauze wipes and pack the wound, as ordered. If a chemical debriding ointment has been ordered, apply it to all exposed areas within the wound, then proceed with packing.
• Cover the packed wound with a nonocclusive dressing.
• Document your findings.

Drainage pouches

Primarily used around wound drains, drainage pouches often are used for excessively draining wounds and fistulas. Ostomy pouches can be used effectively to isolate these wounds and to protect the surrounding skin from maceration if the shape and size of the wound permit pouch application. Many skin barriers and ostomy pouches are available commercially. Follow the manufacturer's directions. Below are some general guidelines:
• Thoroughly cleanse the area surrounding the drainage site.
• Select the type of barrier to be used (Colly-Seel, Karaya, Stomahesive), and follow directions for fitting and application.
• Select an appropriate pouch (preferably drainable), and cut the covered adhesive surface to fit over the wound site. Then remove

the adhesive backing and apply the pouch to the skin barrier.
Clamp the bottom of the pouch.
• Drain the pouch at least once every 8 hours, and record the
amount of drainage on the patient's intake and output sheet.

☐ Burn care

A moderate-to-severe skin burn may be classified as either super-
ficial or deep *partial-thickness* (also known as a second-degree
burn) or *full-thickness* (also known as a third- or fourth-degree
burn), based on its depth and on the postburn presence or absence of deep epithelializing elements—hair follicles and sweat
glands. Less severe (first-degree) burns damage only the epidermis, producing tender, reddened skin as in common sunburn;
they're not considered at length here.

You may be asked to care for a burn patient's wounds by one
of the following methods: cleansing, debridement, application of
topical agents (such as mafenide acetate cream or 1% silver sul-
fadiozine cream), or application of dressings. Some of the most
commonly used techniques in burn care are listed below.

Exposure

This type of burn management minimizes bacterial growth by
decreasing moisture on the skin surface. It involves keeping the
patient in isolation at a controlled temperature of 82° to 84° F.
(27.8° to 28.9° C.). After the burn is exposed to air, antimicrobial
cream is applied at specified intervals. As eschar begins to separate, the necrotic material is trimmed away.

Occlusive dry dressings

This technique, which prevents contractures of the extremities
and increases patient comfort, uses a multilayered-dressing approach. The innermost layer consists of fine mesh gauze that adheres to necrotic debris; the middle layer, bulky roll gauze that
absorbs wound exudate. A stretch bandage is applied on the
outer layer to hold the dressing firmly in place.

Wet dressings

This technique, which also uses a multilayered-dressing approach, can be used during all stages of wound healing. The innermost layer consists of fine mesh gauze used to debride and
encourage granulation. The outer layer consists of multiple layers
of 24-ply gauze pads. The dressing is soaked with various solutions, ranging from normal saline solution to complex antibacterial mixtures.

Single-layer gauze dressings

This technique keeps medication in contact with the wound and
allows for maximum range of motion. It involves application of
antibacterial or antifungal cream (or both) to the burn, which is

then covered with stretch gauze. Absorbent underpads are placed below the dressing to absorb exudate.

Subeschar injection

Ordered especially for infected burns, this technique involves injection of an antimicrobial solution beneath the eschar by hypodermoclysis. After therapy, dressings are then reapplied.

Enzymatic debridement

This technique involves application of a proteolytic enzyme ointment directly to the burn, where it liquefies and degrades necrotic wound protein. A dressing soaked in normal saline solution usually is placed over the ointment.

Skin grafting

This technique, performed when closure may interfere with functioning or is cosmetically undesirable, may be done in the operating room or at the patient's bedside under local anesthesia. A skin graft may be used to prevent infection, allow normal function, or relieve pain.

Various types and sources of grafts may be used, based on the area to be covered and the adequacy of the blood supply to the recipient site. Success in grafting is marked by reestablishing vascularization, which usually takes 3 days to 2 weeks, depending on the thickness of the graft.

Types of grafts include composite, full-thickness, and split-thickness grafts. Composite grafts are composed of skin, subcutaneous tissue, and muscle or bone (or both). Full-thickness grafts include the dermal and epidermal layers of skin. Split-thickness grafts consist of the epidermis and part of the dermal layer.

Both the donor and recipient sites must be scrupulously cleansed and observed for signs of infection or irritation. Follow doctor's orders or hospital policy for preoperative and postoperative care.

Depending on the thickness needed, grafts may be harvested manually or, most commonly, by dermatome. After the graft is smoothed in isotonic solution and positioned in sterile wrapping paper, it is then placed on the recipient site. After positioning, the paper is removed, then the graft is trimmed, stapled or sutured, and dressed.

Temporary, biological dressings may be used. These include homografts, which are taken from cadavers and rejected in 7 to 10 days; heterografts, usually obtained from pigs and rejected in 7 to 10 days; amnion, taken from amnion or chorionic membranes and replaced every 48 hours; and biosynthetic grafts, made of man-made materials and replaced every 3 to 4 days. These grafts may be used together with the patient's own skin and require close observation for signs of infection and rejection (redness, swelling, exudate, drying, and discoloration).

4 Diagnostic Tests

This section includes a listing of some of the most common laboratory and X-ray tests ordered for surgical patients. For detailed information on specific tests ordered for various procedures as well as their nursing implications and interventions, see Section 5.

☐ Laboratory tests

Hematology profile

The body's ability to fight infection, oxygenate tissues, and clot blood (coagulation) is of special concern in the surgical patient. The results of the hematology profile provide a good indication of these parameters. Hematologic tests usually are performed before and after surgery because shifts in blood volume and composition commonly occur.

Note: All tests in the hematologic profile are collected in 7-ml lavender-top tubes containing an anticoagulant. Many of these tests may be done using the same blood sample. Be sure to check with your hospital laboratory.

White blood cell count

This count reflects the number of leukocytes, or white blood cells (WBCs), found in a microliter (cubic millimeter) of whole blood. WBCs usually are counted by a hemacytometer counting chamber called a Coulter counter.

Normal levels

4,100 to 10,900/μl.

Surgical implications

• An elevated WBC count may indicate preoperative or postoperative infection.

• A decreased WBC count may indicate viral infection or a condition that will impair the patient's resistance to infection.

Red blood cell count

This test indicates the number of red blood cells (RBCs) found in a microliter of whole blood. As with WBCs, the test usually is conducted with a Coulter counter.

Normal levels

Males: 4.5 to 6.2 million/μl
Females: 4.2 to 5.4 million/μl

Surgical implications

• An elevated RBC count may indicate dehydration, an important preoperative and postoperative finding.

• A decreased RBC count may suggest anemia, recent hemorrhage, or fluid overload.

Hematocrit level

The hematocrit level measures the percentage of packed RBCs compared with the sera in a whole blood sample. If your patient has a hematocrit level of 35%, this means that a 100-ml whole blood sample contained 35 ml of packed RBCs. RBCs can be packed by centrifuging (spinning) blood collected in a capillary or lavender-top tube. Keep in mind, however, that capillary samples are less accurate and may underestimate the hematocrit level by as much as 5%.

Normal levels
Adult males: 42% to 54%
Adult females: 38% to 46%

Surgical implications
• An elevated hematocrit level may indicate hemoconcentration from fluid loss and suggest dehydration.
• A low hematocrit level may indicate anemia or hemodilution. Hemodilution may suggest compensation for blood loss or fluid overload. Report any level less than 33%.

Hemoglobin level

This test, which measures the number of grams of hemoglobin (oxygen-carrying substance) found in a deciliter (100 ml) of blood, is closely correlated with the patient's RBC count.

Normal levels
Males: 14 to 18 g/dl
Females: 12 to 16 g/dl

Surgical implications
• An elevated hemoglobin level suggests hemoconcentration from fluid loss and dehydration.
• A low hemoglobin level suggests anemia, recent hemorrhage, or fluid retention. Report any level less than 11 g/dl immediately to the surgeon.

Platelet count

This test counts the number of platelets (small oval-shaped blood components that aid coagulation) in a blood sample when the sample is passed through a Coulter counter. When the patient's platelet count is low, most laboratories will do an additional manual count as a routine procedure. In such a case, prepared samples are placed under a microscope with a background grid in the visual field, which enables the technician to count the platelets.

Normal levels
130,000 to 370,000/μl

Surgical implications
• An increased platelet count can result from hemorrhage, recent surgery, or an infectious disorder.
• A decreased count may be caused by a deficiency in folic acid or vitamin B_{12}, pooling of blood in an enlarged spleen, or increased platelet destruction from drugs or an immune disorder.

Erythrocyte sedimentation rate
This test measures the time it takes for erythrocytes to settle at the bottom of a vertical tube when the tube is left standing. Erythrocyte sedimentation rate (ESR), a dependable but nonspecific blood test, often serves as the first indicator of inflammatory disease when other chemical and physical signs may be normal. An abnormal rate indicates the need for further evaluation.

Normal levels
Adult males: 0 to 10 mm/hour
Adult females: 0 to 20 mm/hour

Surgical implications
• An increased ESR can indicate chronic inflammation, autoimmune illness, or anemia.
• A decreased ESR may indicate polycythemia or elevated blood protein levels.

Serum electrolyte levels (chemistry profile)
Electrolytes are chemical substances that, when dissolved, form positively charged particles (cations) and negatively charged particles (anions). The concentration of these various particles in the serum, or extracellular fluid (ECF), is measured in the chemistry profile. Total cations in the ECF should always equal total anion concentration.

Electrolytes are important because they regulate body fluids, maintain acid-base balance, play a role in neuromuscular impulse transmission, and perform other functions related to cellular metabolism.

Electrolyte levels are particularly important in assessing the surgical patient's condition. Elevations or deficiencies in electolyte levels place the patient at risk because such fluctuations affect cardiac functioning, blood volume status, oxygen perfusion capabilities, and immune response.

Because problems related to changes in electrolyte levels may have a rapid onset, you'll need to be familiar with the signs and symptoms of specific problems to ensure the patient receives prompt treatment. Some electrolytes are more important than others; only minor shifts in their concentration can cause the patient serious problems. The most important levels are discussed below.

Note: All samples for the chemistry profile are drawn in 7-ml or 10-ml red-top (clot) tubes. Because these tubes contain no anticoagulant, blood separates or clots in the tube, leaving the serum for evaluation.

Serum potassium levels

The major intracellular cation, potassium (K+) directly affects the functioning of muscles, including the heart. Abnormalities in serum potassium levels are monitored and corrected daily both preoperatively and postoperatively for the following reasons:
• Surgery places increased stress on the cardiovascular system, and changes in electrolyte levels can cause cardiac conduction and contraction abnormalities.
• The surgical patient often requires a nasogastric tube or other tubes that drain fluids containing electrolytes. These electrolytes must be replaced intravenously until the patient can resume his normal diet.
• The surgical procedure itself causes destruction of cells, and potassium (the major intracellular electrolyte) is released into the ECF in proportion to the amount of cellular damage.

Normal levels
3.5 to 5.3 mEq/liter

Surgical implications
Hyperkalemia
An elevated serum potassium level (hyperkalemia) may be the result of substantial tissue damage. The surgical patient may have a mild to high level postoperatively. Elevated levels can cause dangerous cardiac dysrhythmias and should be corrected as soon as they are detected. The body cannot tolerate a substantial deviation from normal levels.

Although a hyperkalemic patient may be asymptomatic, observe for the following signs and symptoms:
• serum potassium levels greater than 5.3 mEq/liter
• areflexia, irritability, weakness, and paresthesia (usually with levels greater than 6.5 mEq/liter)
• bradycardia, dysrhythmias, and tall, peaked T waves on EKG (usually with levels greater than 6.5 mEq/liter)
• abdominal cramping, nausea, and diarrhea (usually with levels greater than 6.5 mEq/liter).

If your patient becomes hyperkalemic, immediately take the following measures:
• Inform your instructor or charge nurse.
• Discontinue all I.V. fluids containing potassium, and replace the fluids with an isotonic solution.
• Discontinue oral potassium supplements.
• Notify the doctor for further orders.

• Place the patient on a bedside monitor or run an EKG if potassium levels are greater than 6.5 mEq/liter.
• Monitor vital signs.
• Document findings and interventions.
   Expect the doctor to order the following for *acute hyperkalemia*:
• calcium chloride I.V. to neutralize toxic neuromuscular effects
• sodium bicarbonate or insulin and glucose I.V. to shift potassium from the ECF to the intracellular fluid (ICF)
• cation exchange resins, such as Kayexalate, to reduce total serum potassium levels.
   Expect the doctor to order the following for *nonacute hyperkalemia*:
• discontinuation of potassium supplements
• restriction of dietary potassium
• oral administration of sodium bicarbonate.
Note: The doctor's choice of treatment depends on the patient's condition and the level of imbalance.

Hypokalemia
Low potassium levels (hypokalemia) are as dangerous as high potassium levels, and the potential for cardiac dysrhythmias is proportionate to the deficiency.
   Hypokalemia may result from various causes. For example, surgical patients may be hypokalemic from previous diuretic therapy, steroid therapy, or renal problems. Patients with gastric distress and decompensation, diarrhea, or vomiting may be hypokalemic from GI losses.
   Although most patients are asymptomatic until potassium levels drop below 2.5 mEq/liter, observe for the following signs and symptoms:
• weakness, hyporeflexia, and paresthesias
• dysrhythmias, increased digitalis sensitivity, orthostatic hypotension, and EKG changes (flattened T waves, presence of U waves, and ST-segment depression)
• anorexia, nausea, and paralytic ileus.
   If your patient is hypokalemic, immediately take the following measures:
• Inform your instructor or the charge nurse.
• Place the patient on a bedside monitor or run an EKG if the potassium level is below 2.5 mEq/liter.
• Notify the doctor for further orders.
   Expect the doctor to order the following:
• oral or I.V. potassium supplements
• cardiac monitoring if the patient's pulse is irregular or the potassium level is below 2.5 mEq/liter.

Serum sodium levels

Sodium (Na^+), the major extracellular cation, affects the amount of total body water, maintains the osmotic pressure of the ECF, and plays a role in transmission of neuromuscular impulses.

Normal levels

135 to 145 mEq/liter

Surgical implications

Hypernatremia

An elevated serum sodium level (hypernatremia) may indicate a state of dehydration caused by water loss. Elevated levels also may result from other disorders, such as impaired renal function. Surgical patients with hypernatremia are considered high risk. (*Note:* When interpreting serum sodium results, you'll need to consider the patient's hydration status.)

Signs and symptoms of hypernatremia include:
• a serum sodium level greater than 145 mEq/liter
• oliguria
• hyporeflexia
• intense thirst
• flushed skin
• dry mucous membranes
• loss of skin turgor and elasticity
• restlessness.

Note: Symptomatic hypernatremia does not occur in patients who can obtain and drink water. These patients will continue to dilute the concentration of sodium in the ECF by responding to the thirst mechanism.

If your patient becomes hypernatremic, immediately take the following measures:
• Report the patient's sodium level immediately to the doctor, your instructor, or the charge nurse.
• Monitor the patient's intake and output.
• Perform neurologic checks every hour (level of consciousness and orientation).
• Administer fluids, if not contraindicated.

Expect the doctor to order the following:
• volume replacement with dextrose 5% in water (for hypernatremia with volume depletion)
• a diuretic followed by dextrose 5% in water (for hypernatremia with volume excess).

Hyponatremia

A decreased serum sodium level (hyponatremia) may result from diuretic therapy, gastric suctioning and decompression (preoperatively or postoperatively), renal insufficiency, a plasma-to-interstitial shift (as in burns or trauma), or decreased sodium intake (rarely).

Signs and symptoms of hyponatremia include:
• anorexia
• nausea
• vomiting
• postural hypotension
• confusion
• coma
• seizures.

If your patient becomes hyponatremic, immediately take the following measures:
• Report the patient's sodium level immediately to the doctor, your instructor, or the charge nurse.
• Monitor the patient's intake and output.
• Obtain urine specific gravity levels.
• Perform neurologic checks every hour.

Expect the doctor to order the following:
• fluid restriction and diuretics (for hyponatremia with volume excess)
• diuretics followed by diuresis with normal saline solution (for hyponatremia with normal ECF volume)
• reexpansion of the ECF with normal saline solution (for hyponatremia with volume depletion).

Serum calcium levels

Calcium (C^+), an extracellular cation important in the transmission of neuromuscular impulses, plays a significant role in intracardiac conduction and myocardial contraction.

Normal levels
8.9 to 10.1 mg/dl

Surgical implications
Hypercalcemia
An elevated calcium level (hypercalcemia) may occur in patients with metastatic carcinoma, multiple fractures, or thyroid disorders and in patients who are chronically immobile. Paget's disease, hyperparathyroidism, and the ingestion of large amounts of antacids also may result in elevated calcium levels.

Signs and symptoms of hypercalcemia include:
• muscular hypotonicity (lack of muscle tone)
• fatigability
• anorexia
• nausea
• vomiting
• dehydration
• central nervous system changes
• constipation
• tremors
• stupor and coma (hypercalcemic crisis).

Note: Because the onset of signs and symptoms is associated with a high mortality, symptomatic patients must receive prompt treatment.

If your patient becomes hypercalcemic, immediately take the following measures:
• Report the patient's calcium level immediately to the doctor.
• Monitor vital signs.
• Perform neurologic checks every hour (every 15 to 30 minutes if abnormal).
• Institute cardiac monitoring if the patient is experiencing changes in level of consciousness or has an irregular pulse.
    Expect the doctor to order the following:
• isotonic saline solution to expand the ECF, increase urine flow, and increase calcium excretion (if the patient's level is greater than 14.5 mg/dl)
• furosemide administration as a method of promoting calcium excretion
• calcitonin administration in patients with impaired renal or cardiovascular function.

Hypocalcemia
Low serum calcium levels (hypocalcemia) may result from renal or thyroid problems, trauma or crush injuries, necrotizing fasciitis, peritonitis, or a primary disorder, such as acute pancreatitis.
    Signs and symptoms of hypocalcemia include:
• stridor and dyspnea
• hyperreflexia
• positive Chvostek's sign
• positive Trousseau's sign (carpopedal spasm)
• abdominal and muscle cramps
• prolonged QT interval on EKG
• tetany.
    If your patient becomes hypocalcemic, immediately take the following measures:
• Report the patient's calcium level immediately to the doctor.
• Check for Chvostek's sign.
• Check for carpopedal spasm.
• Place the patient on seizure precautions if he is symptomatic.
    Expect the doctor to order the following:
• correction of any alkalosis
• administration of calcium chloride or calcium gluconate I.V. in acute cases.

Serum magnesium levels

Next to potassium, magnesium (Mg^+) is the most abundant intracellular cation. It plays an important role in the transmission of neuromuscular impulses; therefore, it can have a profound effect on cardiac muscular function.

Normal levels

1.7 to 2.1 mg/dl (1.5 to 2.5 mEq/liter)

Surgical implications

Hypermagnesemia

An elevated serum magnesium level (hypermagnesemia) usually occurs in patients with renal disease. However, hypermagnesemia may develop in patients with hypovolemia and shock, because magnesium is released from the cells.

Signs and symptoms of hypermagnesemia include:
• tachycardia
• hypotension
• lethargy
• weakness
• EKG changes (widened QRS complex, ST-segment depression, peaked T waves)
• areflexia (in patients with levels greater than 6 mEq/liter)
• somnolence and coma (in patients with levels greater than 10 mEq/liter).

If your patient develops hypermagnesemia, immediately take the following measures:
• Report the patient's magnesium level immediately to the doctor.
• Monitor vital signs every 15 minutes if they are not within normal limits or if the patient's level is above 6 mEq/liter.
• Observe for changes in level of consciousness or orientation; perform neurologic checks every 15 minutes if abnormal.
• Institute cardiac monitoring if the patient is symptomatic or has an irregular pulse.

Expect the doctor to order the following:
• administration of isotonic saline solution I.V. to increase the rate of renal excretion of magnesium
• administration of calcium I.V. to antagonize the neuromuscular actions of magnesium.

Note: The doctor's response will depend on the level of elevation and symptomatology.

Hypomagnesemia

A low serum magnesium level (hypomagnesemia) may result from excessive GI loss from gastric decompression, diarrhea, diuretic therapy, excessive urine loss, burns, or poor dietary intake.

Signs and symptoms of hypomagnesemia include:
• hyperreflexia
• positive Chvostek's sign
• tremors
• delirium
• seizures.

If your patient develops hypomagnesemia, immediately take the following measures:
• Report the patient's magnesium level immediately to the doctor.

• Assess for Chvostek's sign.
• Check the patient's level of consciousness and orientation; if abnormal, perform neurologic checks every 15 minutes.
• Institute cardiac monitoring if the patient's pulse is irregular.
• Institute seizure precautions if the patient is symptomatic.

Expect the doctor to order oral magnesium sulfate or magnesium sulfate I.V. in cases of serious deficiencies (40 to 80 mEq of magnesium per liter of I.V. fluid).

Other parameters

Below is a listing of normal serum levels for other tests that may be included in the chemistry profile:
• Albumin: 3.5 to 5 g/dl
• Alkaline phosphatase:
  —Males: 90 to 240 units/liter
  —Females under age 45: 76 to 196 units/liter
  —Females over age 45: 87 to 250 units/liter
• Bicarbonate: 22 to 34 mEq/liter
• Bilirubin, total: 0.1 to 1 mg/dl
• Blood urea nitrogen: 8 to 20 mg/dl
• Cholesterol: 120 to 330 mg/dl
• Creatinine:
  —Males: 0.8 to 1.2 mg/dl
  —Females: 0.6 to 0.9 mg/dl
• Glucose: 80 to 120 mg/dl
• Total protein: 6.6 to 7.9 g/dl
• Uric acid:
  —Males: 4.3 to 8 mg/dl
  —Females: 2.3 to 6 mg/dl

Arterial blood gas levels

In preoperative patients with chronic respiratory conditions and postoperative patients with respiratory complications, it becomes necessary to evaluate gas exchange at regular intervals by arterial blood gas (ABG) analysis.

ABG samples are drawn by percutaneous arterial puncture with a heparinized syringe or from an arterial line. They must be sent to the laboratory immediately, packed in ice, to prevent further depletion of oxygen by cellular metabolism and, therefore, invalidation of the test.

Normal ranges for ABG levels are as follows:
• PaO_2: 80 to 100 mm Hg
• $PaCO_2$: 35 to 45 mm Hg
• pH: 7.35 to 7.45
• O_2Sat: 95% to 100%
• CO_3^-: 22 to 26 mEq/liter.

See *Acid-base disorders,* page 60, for a list of abnormal ABG findings and their significance.

ACID-BASE DISORDERS

Disorders and arterial blood gas findings	Possible causes	Signs and symptoms
Respiratory acidosis (excess CO₂ retention) pH<7.35 HCO₃⁻>26 mEq/liter (if compensating) Paco₂>45 mm Hg	• Central nervous system depression from drugs, injury, or disease • Asphyxia • Hypoventilation from pulmonary, cardiac, musculoskeletal, or neuromuscular disease	• Diaphoresis, headache, tachycardia, confusion, restlessness, apprehension
Respiratory alkalosis (excess CO₂ excretion) pH>7.45 HCO₃⁻<22 mEq/liter (if compensating) Paco₂<35 mm Hg	• Hyperventilation from anxiety, pain, or improper ventilator settings • Respiratory stimulation from drugs, disease, hypoxia, fever, or high room temperature • Gram-negative bacteremia	• Rapid, deep breathing; paresthesias; light-headedness; twitching; anxiety; fear
Metabolic acidosis (HCO₃⁻ loss, acid retention) pH<7.35 HCO₃⁻<22 mEq/liter Paco₂<35 mm Hg (if compensating)	• HCO₃⁻ depletion from diarrhea • Excessive production of organic acids from hepatic disease, endocrine disorders, shock, or drug intoxication • Inadequate excretion of acids from renal disease	• Rapid, deep breathing; fruity breath; fatigue; headache; lethargy; drowsiness; nausea; vomiting; coma (if severe)
Metabolic alkalosis (HCO₃⁻ retention, acid loss) pH>7.45 HCO₃⁻>26 mEq/liter Paco₂>45 mm Hg (if compensating)	• Loss of hydrochloric acid from prolonged vomiting or gastric suctioning • Loss of potassium from increased renal excretion (as in diuretic therapy) or steroid overdose • Excessive alkali ingestion	• Slow, shallow breathing; hypertonic muscles; restlessness; twitching; confusion; irritability; apathy; tetany; convulsions; coma (if severe)

☐ X-ray tests

Whenever possible, take the opportunity to accompany your patient to any diagnostic X-ray test. By witnessing the test, you will be better prepared to teach other patients about the procedure.

Barium swallow

In this test, the pharynx and esophagus are examined under fluoroscopy after the patient ingests a barium contrast medium. Barium swallow aids in the diagnosis of hiatal hernia, esophageal diverticuli, tumors, ulcers, and varices. The test takes approximately 30 minutes.

Interventions for barium swallow are as follows.

Pre-test
• Explain the test procedure and time schedule to the patient.
• Make sure the patient receives nothing by mouth after midnight on the day of the test.
• Withhold antacids if you suspect reflux; check with the doctor.
• Remove all jewelry and radiopaque objects from the patient.

Post-test
• Allow the patient to resume his usual diet if no further tests are ordered.
• Administer a cathartic, if ordered. If you have not received instructions on administering a cathartic, bring this to the doctor's attention. (Barium is extremely constipating and must be cleared from the GI tract.)

Upper GI and small-bowel series
An upper GI and small-bowel series often is ordered for patients who complain of difficulty swallowing, regurgitation, epigastric pain, or GI bleeding. In this test, the contours of the esophagus, stomach, and small bowel are visualized under fluoroscopy after the patient ingests a barium contrast medium. If necessary, a spot film of suspicious areas may be taken. The test is useful in diagnosing hiatal hernia, diverticuli and varices of the esophagus, stomach ulcers and tumors, regional enteritis, and motility and malabsorption disorders. An upper GI takes approximately 1 hour. A small-bowel follow-through involves a second series of X-rays taken within 3 to 4 hours after the initial test.

Interventions for an upper GI and small-bowel series are as follows.

Pre-test
• Explain the test procedure and time schedule to the patient.
• Make sure the patient receives nothing by mouth after midnight on the day of the test.
• Withhold all oral medications (especially anticholinergics and narcotics) after midnight on the day of the test unless otherwise ordered. (Anticholinergics and narcotics affect intestinal motility, so be sure to check with the patient's doctor.)
• Administer cathartics and enemas according to standing orders or as instructed by the patient's doctor.
• Remove all jewelry and radiopaque objects from the patient.

Post-test
• Explain to the patient that stools may be light colored for 24 to 72 hours after the test.
• Allow the patient to resume his usual diet if no additional tests are ordered.

• Administer a cathartic or enema, as ordered.
• Instruct the patient to notify the nurse if he experiences constipation.

Barium enema and lower GI series

This test involves the visualization of the contours of the large intestine by fluoroscopy after the patient receives an enema of barium sulfate, a radiopaque contrast medium. The test is useful in diagnosing tumors, polyps, diverticula, intestinal obstruction, ulcers, and other GI disorders. A barium enema takes about 1½ hours.

Interventions for a barium enema and lower GI series are as follows.

Pre-test
• Explain the test procedure and time schedule to the patient.
• Administer cathartics and enemas, as ordered, the evening before the test. However, keep in mind the following information:
  —Some conditions, such as GI bleeding, may be a contraindication to routine standing orders for a barium enema preparation on your unit; check with the doctor.
  —When administering enemas for an order that reads "enemas until clear," give no more than three enemas. Inform the surgeon if this is insufficient.
• Administer clear liquids, as ordered, the day before the test or for the evening meal.
• Encourage the patient to drink clear liquids for 12 to 24 hours before the test to ensure adequate hydration.
• Make sure the patient receives nothing by mouth after midnight on the day of the test.

Post-test
• Allow the patient to resume his usual diet if no further tests are ordered.
• Encourage the patient to drink plenty of fluids, because test preparation can cause dehydration.
• Administer a cathartic, as ordered, to clear away any residual barium.
• Explain that stools will be light colored for 24 to 48 hours after test.

Oral cholecystography

Also known as a gallbladder series, an oral cholecystogram involves examination of the gallbladder after the patient ingests iodine tablets (Telepaque), which concentrate in the gallbladder and make it radiopaque to X-rays.

This test can detect gallstones in the gallbladder (cholelithiasis) or in the common bile duct (choledocholithiasis) and aids in the diagnosis of tumors and inflammatory gallbadder disease (cholecystitis).

Interventions for oral cholecystography are as follows.

Pre-test

• Ask the patient if he has any known allergies to iodine dyes or shellfish; report any allergies to the doctor.

• Explain the test procedure and time schedule to the patient.

• Follow the doctor's orders for fat-containing meals or for other special pre-test orders. (Usually, patients are instructed to eat a fat-containing meal at noon, followed by a fat-free meal at dinner, on the day before the test.)

• Make sure the patient receives nothing by mouth after the evening meal on the day before the test.

• Administer six tablets (3 g) of iopanoic acid (most commonly used) 2 to 3 hours after the evening meal, or as ordered.

Post-test

Allow the patient to resume his usual diet after first checking doctor's orders for changes related to any disorders detected by cholecystography.

I.V. pyelography

Also known as excretory pyelography, I.V. pyelography (IVP) involves visualization of structural abnormalities and lesions of the kidneys, ureters, and bladder after administration of a contrast medium I.V.

The contrast medium usually contains iodine and can make the patient feel nauseated, flushed, hot, and otherwise unusual. Feelings of light-headedness, syncope, shortness of breath, and palpitations are indications of a serious, life-threatening reaction and should be reported immediately to the doctor.

Interventions for I.V. pyelography are as follows.

Pre-test

• Ask the patient if he has any known allergies to iodine or shellfish; report any allergies to the doctor.

• Explain the test procedure and time schedule to the patient.

• Make sure the patient receives nothing by mouth for 8 hours before the test.

• Administer a cathartic, if ordered, on the night before the test.

Post-test

• Allow the patient to resume his usual diet if no further tests are ordered.

• Inspect the I.V. site for evidence of hematoma or irritation.

Mammography

Used to detect breast cysts and tumors, especially those not palpable on physical examination, mammography involves placing the breasts (one at a time) between Plexiglas panels and compressing them, then taking X-rays. With the newer-type machines, radiation exposure is minimal.

Mammography also is used to screen for malignant tumors by helping to differentiate cystic palpable lesions from potentially cancerous lesions. A biopsy of suspicious lesions may be necessary to confirm the diagnosis.

Interventions for mammography are as follows.

Pre-test
• Explain the test procedure and time schedule to the patient.
• Instruct the patient to avoid applying powders or lotions on the chest area.
• Remove all jewelry and radiopaque objects from the patient.

Post-test
• Inform the patient when to expect to receive test results. (Check with the doctor.)
• Encourage the patient to ask questions and verbalize anxieties about the procedure and the possible consequences of positive findings. (Discussing concerns may help relieve anxiety by dispelling any misconceptions the patient may have about the test or breast disease. The course of therapy varies with test results. Most lesions are found to be benign.)

Computed tomography

In computed tomography (CT), the patient is placed on an X-ray table that moves through the center of a large machine. As multiple X-ray beams pass through a section of the body, detectors in the CT machine measure the amount of radiation not absorbed by the tissues. (Tissue absorption of radiation varies with tissue density.) A computer reconstructs the information as a three-dimensional image on an oscilloscopic screen. Sectional images can be photographed via an instant camera for a permanent record.

A CT scan can be performed with or without contrast enhancement. In enhanced scans, a contrast medium is injected I.V. to aid in the visualization of specific structures. Different types of CT scans, some of which are listed below, may be performed on various parts of the body.

Biliary tract and liver tomography is used to detect liver neoplasms, abscesses, cysts, and hematomas as well as gallbladder tumors and calculi. It also is used to distinguish obstructive jaundice from nonobstructive jaundice.

Intracranial tomography provides cross-sectional images of various sections of the head. This type of scanning is used to diagnose intracranial tumors, abscesses, hemorrhages, and other brain lesions.

Renal tomography provides cross-sectional views of the kidney. A contrast study enhances the density of the renal parenchyma, helping to differentiate renal masses. Renal tomography is used to detect tumors, obstruction, calculi, polycystic disease, and congenital abnormalities.

Pancreatic tomography usually uses I.V. or oral contrast medium to aid in differentiating tissue densities within the pancreas. The test is used to detect pancreatic neoplasms and distinguish pancreatic disorders from retroperitoneal disorders.

Thoracic tomography, especially useful in detecting minute changes in chest tissue density, is considered one of the most accurate diagnostic tests along with radionuclide scanning. Used to diagnose mediastinal masses, Hodgkin's disease, and thoracic neoplasms, thoracic tomography also is used in differentiating coin-sized lung calcifications from tumors and in distinguishing tumors near the aorta from aortic aneurysm. It also may be used to evaluate metastasis of cancerous lesions to the chest.

Interventions for CT are as follows.

Pre-test

• Ask the patient if he has any known allergies to iodine or shellfish; report any allergies to the doctor.

• Explain the test procedure and time schedule to the patient.

• Tell the patient whether a contrast medium will be used. If contrast medium is to be used, explain that he might experience a flushed, hot sensation or feel slightly unusual while the medium is being injected. Tell him to report any light-headedness, dizziness, shortness of breath, or palpitations immediately, because these could be symptoms of an allergic reaction.

• Make sure the patient receives nothing by mouth for 4 to 6 hours before the test if a contrast medium is to be used.

• If the patient is scheduled for abdominal tests, administer a cathartic the day before the test, as ordered, and make sure he receives nothing by mouth after midnight on the day of the test. If ordered, administer some of the contrast medium orally several hours before the CT scan.

• Obtain a signed consent for the procedure, if one is required.

• Remove all jewelry and other radiopaque objects.

Post-test

• If no contrast medium was used, no interventions are needed.

• If a contrast medium was used, watch for signs and symptoms of delayed hypersensitivity to the dye, including headaches, rashes, and changes in vital signs. (Severe reactions, such as shock, usually occur immediately.)

5 | Quick-Reference Surgical Guidelines

This section reviews some of the common surgical procedures, diagnostic tests, equipment, and emergencies you may encounter on your clinical rotation. Information is presented according to body system. Nursing diagnoses and interventions specific to each surgery are also included. Use these targeted actions along with the general preoperative and postoperative guidelines in Section 2 when working with surgical patients.

☐ Neurologic system

Surgical procedures

Craniotomy. To access the brain for surgery, an opening must be made in the skull. This procedure, called a craniotomy, involves drilling four or five burr holes and cutting the bone between them with a pneumatic drill or Gigli's wire saw. The bone remains attached to the muscle, which acts as a hinge when the flap is turned. Techniques for replacing the flap vary; some surgeons suture the bone flap to the skull with wire through holes drilled in the bone flap.

Transsphenoidal surgery (pituitary). Pituitary surgery to remove tumors may be approached through the sphenoid sinus (as opposed to craniotomy). The incision is made along the interior portion of the nasal septum, so the patient will return from surgery with a bandage over his nostrils (called a mustache dressing or nasal sling).

The posterior pituitary, which stores antidiuretic hormone (ADH), is sometimes damaged in surgery. During the postoperative period, the patient may experience temporary diabetes insipidus (lack of ADH), evidenced by increased urine output and electrolyte imbalances.

Spinal surgery. Spinal cord dysfunction can result from direct trauma, spinal column fractures, tumors, or herniated intravertebral disks. Common spinal surgeries include laminectomy (removing part of the lamina), spinal fusion (solidifying vertebrae by grafting), and chordotomy (dividing the spinothalamic tract to relieve intractable pain).

Preoperative preparation: Craniotomy

Nursing diagnosis

Altered Tissue Perfusion (Cerebral): Decreased Physiologic and Mental Responsiveness related to increased intracranial pressure (ICP)
Desired outcome: The patient will exhibit no signs or symptoms of increased ICP. If signs of increased ICP appear, they will be recognized and reported promptly.

Interventions

1. Perform neurochecks as ordered (see *How to perform a neurocheck,* page 68). Monitor the patient for change in level of consciousness (usually the first sign of increased ICP), bradycardia with an elevated blood pressure or widening pulse pressure, and pupillary size, shape, equality, and response to light.
Rationale: Checking these parameters can warn of possible increased ICP (see *Understanding increased intracranial pressure,* page 69).
2. Assess cranial nerve function (see *Cranial nerve assessment,* page 70).
Rationale: This indicates the condition of the brain stem, which is responsible for maintaining respiration, blood pressure, and consciousness.
3. Notify the doctor if the patient develops a unilaterally fixed, dilated pupil; sudden loss of consciousness; sudden, pronounced changes in vital signs; or sudden onset of a neurologic deficit (such as hemiparesis). Also notify the doctor for onset of abnormal posturing in a patient who is already comatose.
Rationale: These are signs of increased ICP, brain stem compression, or herniation and require immediate treatment by a neurosurgeon.
4. Limit fluids if not contraindicated.
Rationale: This helps to decrease cerebral edema.
5. Monitor ICP.
Rationale: This makes it possible to measure ICP directly and intervene before serious complications occur. (See *Understanding increased intracranial pressure,* page 69, for information on monitoring.)

Nursing diagnosis

Potential for Injury related to loss of motor control secondary to seizures
Desired outcome: The patient's seizures will be medically controlled. If seizures occur, they will be treated promptly, and patient safety will be maintained.

HOW TO PERFORM A NEUROCHECK

Your patient is scheduled for minor surgery. You need to assess his neurologic status, but a complete neurologic examination would be inappropriate. What should you do? Perform a neurocheck. This brief evaluation helps you quickly assess a patient's condition and stability and provides information that may indicate neurologic problems. Neurochecks also are done *routinely* on patients with actual or suspected neurologic problems. Routinely or whenever you note a change in the patient's consciousness level, perform a neurocheck by carefully evaluating the following information:

• *Level of consciousness (LOC).* Does the patient respond when you talk to him, or do you need to apply light pressure on one of his nail beds to get a response? Use the Glasgow coma scale to record your patient's LOC. With each neurocheck, total the response scores. A total of 7 or less indicates a comatose state. An altered consciousness level may be the first indication of increased intracranial pressure (ICP).

• *Vital signs.* Check your patient's pulse rate, blood pressure, and respirations. Altered vital signs may indicate increased ICP or neurogenic shock and will help you identify a hemorrhage or tumor.

• *Pupillary reaction.* Evaluate the patient's direct and consensual response to light. Also, measure his pupil size using a pupil gauge like this:

1 2 3 4 5 6 7

Testing pupillary reaction may help locate a space-occupying brain lesion. Remember, an abnormal pupil reaction occurs on the same side as the lesion (ipsilateral).

• *Motor response.* Test the patient's grip strength, pressure resistance, and ability to move. Evaluating motor response may help locate nerve weakness or damage or a space-occupying lesion. *Note:* Weakness occurs on the side opposite the lesion (contralateral).

Glasgow Coma Scale

By using the Glasgow coma scale below, you can numerically rate your patient's level of consciousness. A total of 7 or less indicates a comatose state.

Test	Reaction score
EYES OPEN	
Spontaneously	4
To speech	3
To pain	2
Not at all	1
VERBAL RESPONSE	
Oriented	5
Confused	4
Inappropriate	3
Incomprehensible	2
None	1
MOTOR RESPONSE	
Obeys commands	5
Localizes pain	4
Flexion to pain	3
Extension to pain	2
None	1

Note: As a general rule, when documenting results, it is better to describe the type of stimulus used as well as the patient's response.

Interventions

Take the following seizure precautions:

1. Keep a soft oral airway or rolled washcloth at the bedside. (This may be inserted during an aura or irritable period, but not once a seizure has started.)

2. Keep emergency drugs, such as I.V. phenytoin and diazepam, readily accessible.

3. Provide a quiet atmosphere.

4. Decrease lighting in the patient's room.

5. Don't allow the patient to smoke unsupervised.

UNDERSTANDING INCREASED INTRACRANIAL PRESSURE

Intracranial pressure (ICP) is the pressure that the intracranial contents exert against the cranial vault. Intracranial contents normally include brain tissue, blood, and cerebrospinal fluid (CSF) and may include hematomas, abscesses, tumors, and fluid surrounding injured tissue (edema). Because the skull is an inflexible vault, if the intracranial contents expand, ICP rises, compressing the brain and causing tissue damage and dysfunction. The skull has only one opening at its base, the foramen magnum. With increased ICP, the brain stem may herniate (push through) this opening. Because the brain stem controls such vital functions as respiration and blood pressure, this complication usually proves fatal.

Assessment
Conduct neurologic checks every 15 to 30 minutes, as ordered, or more frequently if changes are detected. Watch for these signs and symptoms of increased ICP:
• a change in the patient's level of consciousness, including loss of consciousness
• a pupil that dilates or fails to react to light
• pronounced changes in vital signs, especially widening pulse pressure
• sudden onset of signs and symptoms indicating severe neurologic deficit, such as

hemiparesis, hemiplegia, facial paralysis, slurred speech, and abnormal posturing (in a comatose patient).

Prevention or management
To prevent or manage increased ICP, take the following measures:
• Prevent hypercapnia ($PaCO_2 > 45$ mm Hg) and hypoxia ($PaO_2 < 60$ mm Hg).
• Limit the patient's fluid intake, as ordered.
• Position him to avoid neck flexion and head rotation.
• Advise him not to perform Valsalva's maneuver.
• Don't permit long, uninterrupted periods of activity; allow him to rest between nursing procedures.
• Elevate the head of the bed 30 degrees (unless contraindicated).
• Control fever and keep the patient quiet.

Medical interventions
The doctor may initiate ventricular, subarachnoid, or epidural monitoring to detect the earliest signs of increased ICP. To relieve increased ICP in an emergency, he may remove CSF from the ventricles through a small twist-drill hole in the skull, a procedure called ventriculostomy. Keep a ventriculostomy tray at hand, in case of emergency.

---

6. Avoid nonessential procedures.
7. Keep padded bedrails up while the patient is on bed rest.
8. Take no oral temperatures with glass thermometers—rectal temperatures are preferred.
Rationale: These measures provide for patient safety and decrease the activities that may stimulate seizures.

Nursing diagnosis
Knowledge Deficit related to surgical procedure and possible outcomes
Desired outcome: The patient will verbalize preoperative preparation, postoperative care, and possible consequences of craniotomy.

Interventions
1. After the doctor speaks with the patient, discuss surgery with the patient and the family. Encourage questions relating to the entire perioperative period.
Rationale: This helps decrease anxiety and correct any misconceptions the patient or family may have about the procedure and course of recovery.

CRANIAL NERVE ASSESSMENT

To perform a cranial nerve assessment, assess the 12 paired cranial nerves listed below.

Cranial nerve	Assessment
I-Olfactory (Smell)	Have the patient close his eyes. Occlude one nostril with your finger, and ask him to identify nonirritating odors (coffee, cloves, soap, peppermint). Repeat the test on the other nostril.
II-Optic (Vision)	Assess visual acuity with a Snellen chart or newspaper. Or ask the patient to count how many fingers you're holding up. Check visual fields by having the patient sit directly in front of you and stare at your nose. Slowly move your finger from the periphery toward the center until he says he can see it. Check color vision by asking him to name the color of several nearby objects.
III-Oculomotor (Pupillary constriction) **IV-Trochlear** (Upper eyelid elevation; most eye movement) **VI-Abducens** (Downward and inward eye movement; lateral eye movements)	The motor functions of these nerves overlap, so test them together. First, inspect the eyelids for ptosis. Then assess ocular movements by moving your finger to each quadrant of the visual field with the patient's eyes fixed on your finger, and note any eye deviation. Test accommodation and direct and consensual light reflexes.
V-Trigeminal (Sensation to the corneas, nasal and oral mucosa, and facial skin; mastication)	To test motor function, ask the patient to close his jaws tightly. Then try to separate his clenched jaw. Test the corneal reflex by lightly touching the cornea with a cotton wisp. To check sensory function, ask the patient to close his eyes. Then lightly touch his forehead, cheeks, and chin. Can he feel the touch equally on both sides?
VII-Facial (Facial muscles; taste perception)	Have the patient show his teeth, close his eyes against resistance, and puff out his cheeks. Then dab sugar, salt, or vinegar on the front of his tongue. Have him identify these substances by taste.
VIII-Acoustic (Hearing [cochlear]; equilibrium [vestibular])	Rub a few strands of hair between your fingers next to the patient's ear. Then have him identify which ear you selected. Also check his ability to hear a watch ticking or a whisper. Observe the patient's balance. Does he sway when walking or standing?
IX-Glossopharyngeal (Swallowing and phonation; sensation to the pharyngeal, soft palate, and tonsillar mucosa; taste perception; salivation) **X-Vagus** (Swallowing and phonation; sensation to the exterior ear's posterior wall and behind the ear; sensation to the thoracic and abdominal viscera)	First, have the patient identify tastes at the back of his tongue. Then inspect the soft palate. Observe for symmetrical elevation when the patient says *aah.* Touch the soft palate's mucous membrane with a swab to elicit the palatal reflex. Touch the posterior pharyngeal wall with a tongue depressor to elicit the gag reflex.
XI-Spinal accessory (Uvula and soft palate movement; movement of sternocleidomastoid and trapezius muscle)	Palpate and inspect the sternocleidomastoid muscle as the patient pushes his chin against your hand. Palpate and inspect the trapezius muscle as the patient shrugs his shoulders against your resistance. Also have the patient stretch out his hands toward you.
XII-Hypoglossal (Tongue movements involved in swallowing and speech)	Observe the tongue for asymmetry, atrophy, deviation to one side, and fasciculations. Ask the patient to push his tongue against a tongue depressor. Then have him move his tongue rapidly in and out and from side to side.

2. Take the family or significant other to visit the intensive care unit the day before surgery if you feel it is appropriate. Respect the family's decision if they elect not to go.

Rationale: Many patients return from the recovery room with equipment—such as tubes, ventilators, or intracranial monitors—that can be frightening to the family at first sight. Ask an experienced nurse about the equipment your patient is likely to have postoperatively. Have her accompany you and the family should they decide to make the preoperative visit.

Postoperative care: Craniotomy

Nursing diagnosis

Altered Tissue Perfusion (Cerebral): Decreased Physiologic and Mental Responsiveness related to increased intracranial pressure (For desired outcome and interventions, see "Preoperative preparation: Craniotomy" above.)

Nursing diagnosis

Potential for Injury related to loss of motor control secondary to seizures

(For desired outcome and interventions, see "Preoperative preparation: Craniotomy" above.)

Nursing diagnosis

Potential for Infection related to leakage of cerebrospinal fluid (CSF) from the surgical site

Desired outcome: The dressing will remain dry; any signs of CSF leakage will be reported.

Interventions

1. Check dressing every hour for 24 hours for signs of CSF drainage—blood encircled by a yellowish ring (halo sign)—and promptly report such findings to the doctor. Then, reinforce dressing.

Rationale: Leaking CSF provides a direct route for bacteria to invade the brain and cause life-threatening infections.

2. Observe for CSF drainage from the nose or ears. Check nose drainage with a Dextrostix. CSF is positive for glucose; mucus is not. Promptly report positive findings.

Rationale: Leaking CSF provides a direct route for bacteria to invade the brain and cause life-threatening infections.

Nursing diagnosis

Ineffective Breathing Pattern related to cerebral or brain stem compression secondary to cerebral edema

Desired outcome: Altered breathing patterns will be identified and reported immediately.

Interventions
1. Monitor the patient's respiratory rate, depth, and rhythm. Abnormal patterns include:
• Cheyne-Stokes respirations (a rhythmic waxing and waning of both rate and depth of respiration alternating with short periods of apnea)
• central neurogenic hyperventilation (sustained, regular hyperpnea with forced inspiration and expiration)
• apneustic breathing (prolonged gasping inspiration followed by brief, inefficient expiration)
• cluster breathing (irregular breathing alternating with periods of apnea)
• ataxic breathing (completely irregular breathing, typically progressing to apnea).
Rationale: These respiratory patterns are ominous signs that indicate deterioration of brain stem function.
2. Monitor arterial blood gases (ABG) levels and report abnormalities. Normal values: pH = 7.35 to 7.45, $PaCO_2$ = 35 to 45 mm Hg, PaO_2 = 80 to 100 PaO_2 mm Hg.
Rationale: Decreased ventilation leads to hypercapnia and hypoxia.

Preoperative preparation: Spinal surgery

Nursing diagnosis
Knowledge Deficit related to surgery and postsurgical care
Desired outcome: The patient will verbalize an understanding of the surgical procedure and procedures associated with the postoperative period.

Interventions
1. Discuss preoperative procedures and postoperative care with the patient and family or significant other. Ask the patient or family to state what they know about the procedure and possible outcomes.
Rationale: The patient may have unrealistic expectations about the surgery, such as complete pain relief. Also, the patient should know about possible consequences of surgery, such as bladder or bowel incontinence.
2. Show the patient the logrolling procedure, and practice it.
Rationale: This will facilitate turning postoperatively, especially in the immediate postoperative period, and will prevent injury.
3. Discuss any special braces, beds, or other devices that will be used postoperatively.
Rationale: It is frightening to awaken from anesthesia restricted by a brace, in a turning frame, or surrounded by other unfamiliar equipment.

Postoperative care: Spinal surgery

Nursing diagnosis

Potential for Injury: Spinal Cord Damage related to postoperative spinal misalignment

Desired outcome: Spinal alignment will be maintained at all times. No injury to the spinal cord or vertebrae will occur.

Interventions

1. Logrolling (if ordered). This procedure requires at least three trained people. The patient should have a turning sheet on the bed. The object is to turn the patient while keeping his spine properly aligned at all times. On the count of three, one person turns the patient's head, another the trunk, and another the legs simultaneously. The people stationed at the trunk and legs use the gathered edges of the turning sheet. Support the patient in this position with foam wedges and pillows.

2. Turning with skeletal traction (skeletal tongs). Logroll the patient, with one person responsible for turning the patient's head in alignment with the body. Use foam wedges or pillows to support the back and prevent the patient from rolling back to a flat position. If maintaining horizontal alignment of the cervical spine is a problem, support the patient's head with a pillow when turning him. Be sure that traction weights hang freely at all times and that tongs are tightened periodically by the doctor to prevent accidental disengagement.

Note: If skeletal tongs come off, immediately evaluate the patient's level of consciousness and assess him for any new neurologic deficits. Place sandbags on each side of the supine patient's head to immobilize the cervical spine, and tell him not to move. Notify the doctor immediately; then stay with the patient.

3. Using turning frames or CircOlectric beds. Depending on the frame, one or two people will be required to turn the patient. Before you assist, read the manufacturer's directions thoroughly, state the procedure to your supervising nurse, and have your instructor or a trained nurse present. Remember to position the padding appropriately and free all traction weights, indwelling catheters, tubes, or other equipment to avoid entanglement during the turning procedure.

Rationale: All these devices and interventions help ensure spinal alignment and protect the patient from misalignment complications, such as additional neurologic deficits, spinal cord compression or severance, and vertebral injury.

Diagnostic tests

Angiography, cerebral. The purpose of this study is to locate cerebrovascular abnormalities, such as tumors, cerebrovascular anomalies, hemorrhage, or aneurysms. The patient's carotid artery is injected with dye medium via a cannula, and a series of cerebrovascular X-rays is obtained.

Brain scan, radioisotope. This test diagnoses masses, vascular lesions, or ischemic or infarcted areas of the brain. A bolus of radionuclide is injected into the brachial vein. Rapid X-rays are taken to follow the isotope through the brain. A scanner shows images that may reveal pathologic abnormalities in tissue or blood flow.

Brain stem auditory evoked response (BAER). This test evaluates the eighth cranial nerve, thought to be one of the last portions of the brain stem to remain intact in cases of severe brain stem deterioration. Most often administered to comatose or obtunded patients, the test doesn't require the patient's cooperation. An electrode is placed deep in the ear canal, and surface electrodes record electrical evoked responses, which appear as electric sequelae on computer-averaged EEGs.

Computed tomography (CT) scan, cerebral. This test is used to diagnose intracranial lesions, evaluate extent of intracranial injury, and monitor effects of chemotherapy and radiotherapy. The patient lies immobile on a table, with his head stationary inside the scanner. X-rays are taken at 1-degree intervals in a 180-degree arc. Contrast medium is injected (if ordered) and a new series of X-rays taken.

Digital subtraction angiography (DSA), cerebral. This study is used to visualize cerebral blood flow and detect vascular abnormalities, such as aneurysms, tumors, and hematomas. A type of I.V. angiography, DSA combines X-ray methods and a computerized subtraction technique with fluoroscopy to visualize brain structures without interference from bone or soft tissue.

Echoencephalography, cerebral. This study determines the position of midline cerebral structures. A transducer, placed on the temporal area, emits an ultrasonic beam that reflects off midline brain structures, giving evidence of distance from transducer to structure. The study has largely been replaced by the CT scan.

Electroencephalography. This study, which evaluates the brain's electrical activity in various neurologic disorders, is used to determine the presence and type of epilepsy. Electrodes (usually flat, but may be needle electrodes) are placed on the scalp. A machine records electrical brain activity while the patient is lying down or sitting in a reclining chair.

Electromyography. This study helps differentiate muscle disease from nervous disorders and aids in diagnosing neuromuscular disorders, such as myasthenia gravis. Needle electrodes are placed in muscles to be tested. The muscles' electrical signals are then recorded during rest and contraction.

Lumbar puncture. A lumbar puncture is used to measure CSF pressure and to obtain CSF specimens for laboratory investigation. The test is usually performed while the patient is in bed. Position the patient on his side, with his back at the edge of the bed. Help him maintain a knee-to-chest position throughout the procedure by placing one arm around his knees and the other around his neck. The proposed puncture site (usually between the third and fourth lumbar vertebrae) is prepared, draped, and anesthetized using 1% or 2% lidocaine. The needle is inserted and the stylet removed. A manometer with a stopcock is attached to the needle, and CSF pressure is measured. (Normal CSF pressure is 50 to 180 mm H_2O.) The stopcock is opened and specimens are collected. Containers are labeled 1, 2, and 3 in order. Another pressure measurement is taken, and the needle is removed. An adhesive bandage is placed on the site.

Magnetic resonance imaging (MRI). This test images the brain's anatomy to diagnose tumors, infarcts, vascular malformations, and other abnormalities. The patient is placed under a strong magnetic field and pulsed with a radio frequency. The body's soft tissue releases its own radio frequency waves; these are recorded, and an image is developed.

Equipment, tubes, and drains

Halo traction vest. Halo traction immobilizes the cervical vertebrae after surgery. The halo traction vest, unlike skeletal tongs, allows the patient to ambulate. Notify the doctor if the vest or pins become dislodged or misaligned or if the patient has a sudden motor or sensory loss.

Cleanse pin sites every 4 hours with hydrogen peroxide on cotton-tipped applicators. Evaluate for "tenting" of skin around the sites, remove crusts, check drainage, and watch for loosening or movement of pins. Unless contraindicated, apply povidone-iodine dressings to the sites if they appear infected. Wash the patient's chest and back daily (reach these areas by loosening the vest's Velcro straps). Dry the areas thoroughly, preferably with a hair dryer on cool setting. Observe for reddened pressure areas.

ICP monitoring devices. ICP monitoring measures the pressure that intracranial contents exert against the skull. Three types of ICP monitoring devices are the ventricular catheter, the subarachnoid screw, and the epidural sensor.

In ventricular catheterization, a silicone rubber catheter is inserted into the lateral ventricle through a drill hole in the skull. The apparatus is connected to a pressurized flush system and transducer. Although this method measures ICP most accurately, it also carries the greatest risk of infection.

The subarachnoid screw is a catheter that's inserted into the subarachnoid space through a drill hole in the skull. The apparatus is connected to a pressurized flush system and transducer. Placing this screw is easier than placing a ventricular catheter and carries less risk to the patient, but large amounts of CSF can't be drained off as with ventricular catheterization.

The epidural sensor is a fiber-optic sensor inserted through a drill hole into the epidural space. This method carries the least risk to the patient, but because it measures ICP indirectly (pressure of dura against the skull), it is also the least accurate monitoring method.

Jackson-Pratt drain. Placed in the subdural space during craniotomy, this drain is an oval, clear, pliable reservoir connected to drain tubing. The drain is usually left in place for 24 to 48 hours after surgery. Empty and record output at least every 8 hours. Open the cap and drain the contents from the bulb using sterile procedure. Compress the bulb fully and reclose the cap to re-establish suction.

Skull tongs. Skull tongs are used in cervical skeletal traction to immobilize the spine and maintain vertebral alignment. This prevents damage to the spinal cord from unstable vertebral bone fragments or misaligned vertebrae. Commonly used tongs include Crutchfield, Gardner-Wells, and Vinke.

Emergencies

Coma (sudden onset). Coma is a state of unconsciousness from which the patient, unresponsive to verbal or painful stimuli, can't be aroused. Some classify coma as moderate or deep (mild response vs. no response). Sudden onset of coma is usually attributed to neurologic factors, although secondary conditions, such as diabetes or drug overdose, may also result in loss of consciousness. Sudden onset of coma is an ominous sign indicating deterioration of the ascending reticular activating system (ARAS) that forms part of the brain stem. The ARAS is responsible for alertness; the brain stem, for such vital life processes as respiration and blood pressure. When damage occurs to the ARAS or brain stem, the patient's life is threatened.

Signs and symptoms include the following:
• no response to pain or verbal stimuli
• pupillary changes (vary with cause)
• possible abnormal breathing pattern and decreased blood pressure
• decorticate posturing (characterized by a rigid spine, inwardly flexed arms, extended legs, and plantar flexion; may indicate a lesion at the level of the diencephalon) or decerebrate posturing

(characterized by a rigid and possibly arched spine, rigidly extended arms and legs, and plantar flexion; may indicate a brain stem lesion).

Expect to do the following:

• Establish and maintain patent airway.

—Insert an oropharyngeal airway immediately. Prepare to intubate if ventilatory problems develop. Administer oxygen at 8 liters/minute until the doctor arrives.

—Place the patient on his side, and suction his mouth, if necessary, to clear the airway.

• Perform a neurologic assessment.

—Check the patient's pupils for size, shape, equality, reaction to light, and deviation.

—Monitor the patient's vital signs.

—Evaluate the depth of coma, using the Glasgow coma scale on page 68.

Expect the doctor to do the following:

• Perform a neurologic examination.

• Obtain ABG measurements, and intubate if impaired ventilation is clinically apparent.

• Place the patient on a cardiac monitor.

• Order a CT scan.

• Rule out postictal (postseizure) state.

• Order laboratory studies to rule out hypoglycemia.

• Perform a brief physical examination and order laboratory studies to rule out internal bleeding.

• Rule out accidental drug overdose.

• Rule out hypovolemia.

Note: Sudden loss of consciousness in neurosurgical patients is frequently caused by increased ICP from hemorrhage, edema, injury, or other space-occupying lesions. This results in compression and herniation of parts of the brain that sustain consciousness, rendering the patient comatose.

Seizures, status epilepticus. Seizures, which are caused by irritable brain tissue that may be idiopathic or the result of injury, surgery, or a space-occupying lesion, are primarily classified as partial or generalized.

Partial seizures can be classified as simple (focal) or complex (temporal lobe or psychomotor). Simple partial seizures can be motor, sensory, or autonomic—the most common being motor (jacksonian) seizures, which involve localized clonic jerking of a muscle group that sometimes progresses in an orderly fashion to other parts of the body (jacksonian march). Complex partial seizures involve impairment of consciousness, thinking, and behavior.

Generalized seizures, which occur without focal onset, are characterized by loss of consciousness, tonic-clonic rigidity, incontinence, and increased salivation. The patient may even cry out at the seizure's onset.

An absence (petit mal) seizure is a type of generalized seizure characterized by a sudden loss of awareness (usually without motor symptoms) but not a loss of consciousness. During the seizure, which usually lasts from 10 to 30 seconds, the patient appears to stare blankly and his breathing and motor functions appear normal; normal activity stops and resumes without his awareness. Although these attacks occur primarily in children, adults should be cautioned not to operate potentially dangerous equipment because the attacks can occur at any time.

Seizures generally progress through several phases: prodromal, aura, ictal, and postictal. During the prodromal phase, the patient may experience mood or behavioral changes. During the aura phase—a state of altered consciousness that often precedes a focal seizure and lasts from a few seconds to about 5 minutes—the patient stares blankly and may experience psychosensory or psychomotor hallucinations, such as foul smells or tastes, vertigo, and unfamiliarity with his environment. The ictal phase marks the period of full seizure activity. The postictal phase is a period of slow recovery during which the patient may experience altered levels of consciousness, fatigue, and confusion.

Before, during, and after a seizure, observe and document the following:
• Before the seizure (prodromal): What was the patient's level of consciousness? What was he doing before the attack? In what part of the body did the seizure start?
• During the seizure (ictal): Did the patient cry out? Did he display automatisms, such as eye fluttering or lip smacking? Were his movements bilateral? How long did the seizure last? Did you note increased salivation, cyanosis, or incontinence? How would you describe his pupillary reactions?
• After the seizure (postictal): Did the patient appear lethargic or confused? Did he complain of headaches? Did you note any speech impairment or other neurologic deficits, such as transient hemiplegia?

During a seizure, expect to do the following:
• Support the patient's head.
• Lower him to the floor if he is standing at the seizure's onset.
• Insert a soft oropharyngeal airway before the full onset of the seizure.
• Maintain the patient's airway and oxygenation.
• Observe and report the event as indicated above.
• Administer medication, as ordered.

• Reorient the patient and perform a neurologic assessment after the seizure.

For all patients susceptible to brain irritability and therefore seizures, take the following precautions to ensure safety during an attack:

• Place the patient in a private, carpeted room, if possible.
• Keep a soft oropharyngeal airway or rolled washcloth on the bed's headboard. Insert this in the patient's mouth if he is experiencing restlessness or an aura that may precede a seizure. *Note:* Never insert an airway once the seizure is in progress.
• Keep the bed in a low position, and be sure the side rails are padded and up while the patient is in bed.
• Maintain a quiet environment.
• Never take the patient's temperature orally.

Status epilepticus, a medical emergency, consists of continuous tonic-clonic seizure activity without complete recovery between seizures. Signs and symptoms include possible unconsciousness, continuous tonic-clonic activity, sustained eye deviation, incontinence, diaphoresis, labored breathing with periods of apnea, and cyanosis.

Prolonged seizure activity results in hypoxia, hypoglycemia, and hyperthermia. These conditions lead to continuing seizure activity that, if untreated, eventually results in metabolic and physical exhaustion and death.

Expect to do the following for a patient in status epilepticus:
• Maintain adequate oxygenation while medically treating the patient. (Hypoxia is the greatest physiologic danger. Brain damage and death may ensue if adequate oxygen is not supplied.)
—Turn the patient's head to the side, and suction if necessary during less active intervals.
—Obtain ABG measurements when possible.
—Administer oxygen at 8 to 10 liters/minute.
—Assist with intubation during the postictal phase. (Intubation through the nasal route may be attempted.)
• Protect the patient from injury.
—Hold the patient's head.
—Lower the patient to the floor if he is standing at the seizure's onset.
—Administer anticonvulsants, such as diazepam I.V. push; repeat two or three times at 20-minute intervals, under supervision, as ordered. (Besides diazepam, medications commonly used to treat seizures include phenytoin, phenobarbital, and paraldehyde.)
• Insert a nasogastric tube, as ordered, once the patient is intubated.

☐ Respiratory system

Surgical procedures

The most common pulmonary surgeries are pneumonectomy (removal of a lung), lobectomy (removal of a lobe), segmental resection or segmentectomy (removal of one or more lung segments), and wedge resection (removal of a small localized area, or wedge, on the surface of the lung).

Exploratory thoracotomy is performed to examine the lung for evidence of suspected lung cancer or other surgically correctable pulmonary diseases.

Preoperative preparation

Nursing diagnosis

Altered Respiratory Function related to pulmonary disease
Desired outcome: The patient will have optimal ventilation and perfusion at the time of surgery.

Interventions

1. Assess the patient for level of ventilatory and pulmonary impairment.
Rationale: This evaluation will become the data base for your preoperative care plan.
2. Force fluids (at least 2,500 ml/day) if not contraindicated.
Rationale: Fluids help to liquefy bronchopulmonary secretions.
3. Encourage pulmonary hygiene with mobility, coughing, and deep breathing at least every hour while patient is awake.
Rationale: This is the most effective method of clearing the bronchial airways and preventing stasis of secretions.
4. Auscultate breath sounds every 2 hours; suction if you hear coarse crackles over the large bronchi and the patient isn't able to clear sounds by coughing.
Rationale: Course crackles indicate mucus in the large airways, which obstructs ventilation. Suctioning helps remove mucus and causes the patient to cough and expel secretions on his own. Don't suction if the patient can cough and expel his own secretions.
5. Administer respiratory therapy under supervision, as ordered, in the absence of a respiratory therapist.
Rationale: Special treatments help to liquefy mucous secretions (nebulization) and expand the alveolar spaces to increase ventilation. (See "Incentive spirometer" and "Intermittent positive-pressure breathing", page 86.)
6. Advise the patient not to smoke throughout the perioperative period.
Rationale: Smoking decreases oxygen saturation of the blood and increases mucus production.

Nursing diagnosis

Altered Nutrition: Less than Body Requirements related to high caloric expenditure from chronic lung disease
Desired outcome: The patient will maintain body weight.

Interventions

1. Administer a high-calorie, high-protein diet. Ask the dietitian for supplements if needed.
Rationale: Surgery is a catabolic process. Also, patients with obstructive lung disease need more calories to maintain labored breathing.
2. Notify the doctor if the patient loses any weight while in the hospital.
Rationale: The preoperative nutritional goal is to supplement the patient to an anabolic state and maintain his weight throughout the perioperative period.

Nursing diagnosis

Potential for Infection related to impaired skin integrity of proposed surgical site
Desired outcome: The proposed incision site will remain free from infection or irritation.

Interventions

1. Keep the operative site clean with antibacterial scrubs.
Rationale: This prevents bacterial growth and has a lasting cumulative bacteriostatic action.
2. Report any lesions, rashes, or skin irritation at or near the proposed surgical site.
Rationale: Any of the above problems may be a reason to postpone the surgery.

Nursing diagnosis

Knowledge Deficit related to the surgical preparation, procedure, and recovery
Desired outcome: The patient will verbalize an understanding of perioperative events and will demonstrate independence in performing postoperative exercises.

Interventions

1. Discuss the doctor's explanation of the surgical procedure.
Rationale: Patients may have misconceptions of what is involved in the surgery or unrealistic expectations about the outcome.
2. Have the patient practice postoperative breathing exercises.
Rationale: This helps to clear the lungs preoperatively and familiarize the patient with the postoperative pulmonary regimen.
3. Have the patient visit the intensive care unit (ICU) if he is to return there after surgery. Explain the major equipment that will be used postoperatively.

Rationale: Knowing what to expect decreases the panic associated with waking up in the ICU environment. Have an experienced nurse accompany you if the patient wishes to make the preoperative visit.

4. Review all forms of respiratory therapy that will be used throughout the perioperative period.

Rationale: Being familiar with the purpose of respiratory equipment and therapy usually increases compliance and decreases associated anxiety.

5. Explain the purpose of closed chest drainage and how it will influence immediate postoperative activity. Let the patient know he will be expected to turn, cough, deep-breathe, and sit up with the tubes in place, and that these activities will not influence chest tube function.

Rationale: Patients tend to remain immobile because of fear and pain associated with chest tubes.

6. Tell the patient he won't be able to talk during the immediate postoperative period because of an endotracheal tube that will remain in place. Establish an alternate means of communication.

Rationale: Being unable to communicate basic needs postoperatively is very distressing, especially if the patient doesn't anticipate this.

7. Explain to the patient the purpose of endotracheal suctioning.

Rationale: Endotracheal suctioning is uncomfortable and frightening. Some patients panic from the feeling of suffocation if they are not informed beforehand about the procedure and the need to maintain a clear airway.

Postoperative care

Nursing diagnosis

Impaired Gas Exchange related to decreased lung surface, atelectasis, and splinting from incisional pain

Desired outcome: The patient's ABG levels will be normal, and no impaired gas exchange will be evident.

Interventions

1. Monitor ABG levels.

Rationale: Increased $PaCO_2$ (>50 mm Hg) and decreased PaO_2 (<50 mm Hg) indicate inadequate ventilation.

2. Auscultate breath sounds every 2 hours.

Rationale: Coarse crackles over the major bronchi indicate a need to clear the airway by having the patient cough or by endotracheal suctioning. Fine crackles indicate fluid accumulation in the alveoli and smaller airways.

3. Position the patient according to the type of surgery. Help him to become as comfortable as possible.

Rationale: Some surgeries, such as pneumonectomy, require special positioning (for example, not lying on the surgical site until ordered). If the patient is uncomfortable, his breathing rate, depth, and pattern will be affected.

Nursing diagnosis

Ineffective Respiratory Pattern related to pain or sedation
Desired outcome: The patient will have a normal respiratory pattern.

Interventions

1. Observe the patient's chest for respiratory rate, depth, and pattern.
Rationale: Shallow breathing with less than 14 breaths/minute or more than 25 breaths/minute or an irregular breathing pattern can result in hypoventilation.
2. Decrease sedation if the patient's respiratory rate, depth, or pattern is negatively affected.
Rationale: Decreased respiratory rate or depth or an irregular respiratory pattern can result in hypoventilation.

Nursing diagnosis

Ineffective Airway Clearance related to mucus obstruction
Desired outcome: The patient will have a clear, patent airway and perform pulmonary hygiene independently.

Interventions

1. Auscultate breath sounds every 2 hours; suction as needed.
Rationale: Suctioning clears the major airways of mucus and increases ventilation.
2. Hyperventilate the patient before suctioning. Use an Ambu bag with 100% oxygen, administering breaths at regular intervals for 1 minute.
Rationale: This helps prevent hypoxia associated with suctioning.

Nursing diagnosis

Altered Respiratory Pattern related to postoperative tension pneumothorax
Desired outcome: The patient will show no evidence of a tension pneumothorax. If the patient does develop a tension pneumothorax, it will be promptly assessed and reported.

Interventions

1. Observe respiratory rate, depth, and pattern.
Rationale: Restricted breathing could indicate a buildup of pressure within the chest. This happens when air leaks from the lung incision and becomes trapped in the chest.
2. Auscultate the chest for mediastinal shift. If you hear tracheal breath sounds to the right or left of the midline, report this condition to the doctor.

Rationale: If a large amount of air becomes trapped in one side of the chest cavity, it will push the heart, trachea, and mediastinum in the opposite direction from the midline.

3. Check the patient's chest and suture line for subcutaneous emphysema. This presents as a crackling feeling when you palpate the skin.

Rationale: Internal leakage from the lung incision can cause air to infiltrate surface tissues.

Nursing diagnosis

Fluid Volume Deficit related to postoperative hemorrhage

Desired outcome: The patient will not hemorrhage postoperatively. If he should hemorrhage, it will be detected and reported immediately.

Interventions

1. Check chest tubes for drainage of bright-red blood. Normal bloody drainage is usually brownish red.

Rationale: Bright-red blood can indicate the beginning of acute bleeding from the internal surgical incision.

2. Check volume of output from chest tubes every hour during the immediate postoperative period. Report drainage exceeding 100 ml/hour or 50 ml/hour for 4 hours.

Rationale: Rapid accumulation of bloody drainage may indicate hemorrhage.

3. Observe the patient for decreased blood pressure, tachycardia, cool extremities, decreased level of consciousness, diaphoresis, and decreased urine output.

Rationale: These are signs and symptoms of hemorrhagic shock and should be reported immediately.

Nursing diagnosis

Decreased Tissue Perfusion (Pulmonary): Ischemia or Infarction of Lung Tissue related to pulmonary embolus (PE)

Desired outcome: The patient will not develop PE.

Interventions

1. Observe the patient for complaints of chest pain; shortness of breath; frothy, pink-tinged sputum; decreased blood pressure; and sudden increased anxiety. Notify your instructor, supervising nurse, or the doctor if you suspect PE.

Rationale: These are signs and symptoms associated with acute PE.

2. Auscultate breath sounds if PE is suspected.

Rationale: Localized wheezing may be present over the affected lung area.

3. Monitor ABG levels.

Rationale: ABG measurements usually reflect decreased PaO_2.

Diagnostic tests

Bronchoscopy. In this study, a flexible or rigid bronchoscope is used to inspect the trachea and bronchi. Looking through the bronchoscope into the bronchial lumen, the doctor can detect bleeding sites, assess resectability of tumors, remove foreign objects (with the rigid scope), and evaluate other pathologic processes. Cultures, biopsies, and bronchial washings also can be performed with the bronchoscope.

Chest X-ray. Chest radiography reveals the location and size of a lesion and identifies structural abnormalities that influence ventilation and perfusion. For example, a chest X-ray can determine pneumothorax, fibrosis, atelectasis, and infiltrates.

Pulmonary angiography. This diagnostic test permits examination of pulmonary circulation. After a catheter is inserted into the pulmonary artery, a contrast dye is injected, and a series of X-rays are taken to detect blood flow abnormalities. This study can aid in diagnosing pulmonary emboli and infarction and provides more reliable results than the ventilation-perfusion scan.

Thoracic CT scan. The CT scan provides a three-dimensional image of the lung to assess for abnormalities in tracheal or bronchial configuration, defines lesions (such as tumors or abscesses), and defines abnormal lung shadows. A contrast study can highlight blood vessels to achieve greater discrimination.

Ventilation-perfusion scan (lung scan). Although less reliable than pulmonary angiography, this test carries fewer risks to the patient. The test can evaluate ventilation and perfusion defects, detect pulmonary emboli, and evaluate pulmonary function. A contrast study, it requires injecting a radioactive contrast dye before scanning.

Equipment, tubes, and drains

Chest tubes, closed drainage systems. The two- or three-bottle closed chest drainage system has been replaced in most hospitals with a disposable one-piece plastic drainage unit, such as Pleur-Evac or Argyle. These units protect the patient from hazards associated with breakable bottles, reflux of drainage into the chest, inaccurate suction, and air leaks. The principle of the disposable unit, however, is the same as the bottle system.

Endotracheal (ET) tubes. An ET tube provides a rigid, patent airway through the mouth or nose into the trachea. It is used during lengthy surgical procedures, in cases of respiratory failure or arrest, or when relatively long-term ventilatory assistance is anticipated. ET tubes are cuffed and come in various sizes. For the adult female, size 7 or 8 is usually adequate; sizes 8, 9, and (rarely) 10 are used to intubate adult males.

Incentive spirometer. This device provides positive feedback for the patient by allowing him to gauge his progress at producing maximum inspiration. When the patient inspires, the incentive spirometer responds by lighting up the inspired volume level or by lifting balls within a closed plastic compartment. Unlike regular deep-breathing exercises, incentive spirometry provides tangible evidence of the patient's effort. The device is used to prevent atelectasis by expanding the alveoli during inspiration. For incentive spirometry to be effective, the patient must hold his breath at the end of inspiration for 3 seconds. This procedure should be done three times each hour, with each session lasting 10 minutes.

Intermittent positive-pressure breathing (IPPB). The purpose of IPPB is to expand the alveoli for better gas exchange, improve ventilation-perfusion ratios, loosen tenacious secretions, and distend the tracheobronchial tree, lowering airflow resistance and reducing the effort needed to breathe effectively. The IPPB machine accomplishes this by delivering a mixture of air and oxygen to the lungs at a preset pressure. IPPB treatments last 10 to 20 minutes and are given three or four times daily, usually by respiratory therapists. You should explain the purpose of IPPB to your patient before surgery because this tends to increase his compliance postoperatively.

Oximeter. An oximeter continuously monitors oxygenation by means of a sensing device placed on the patient's earlobe, finger, or toe. The sensor transmits signals to a bedside oximeter unit. Oximetry can detect a change in the patient's oxygenation status within 6 seconds by monitoring transmission of light waves through the earlobe's vascular bed. The oximeter is not recommended for use on patients with severely impaired peripheral circulation. For these patients, a special nasal probe is provided.

Oxygen delivery systems. These systems include a nasal cannula, a simple face mask, a partial rebreather mask, a non-rebreather mask, and a Venturi mask. The patient's needs determine which method to choose. For more information, see *Evaluating common oxygen delivery systems.*

Tracheostomy tubes. A tracheostomy tube provides a rigid, patent airway directly into the trachea and is used primarily for patients who require long-term ventilation or for unconscious or paralyzed patients who would have trouble maintaining a patent airway. Tracheostomy tubes are plastic or metal (the latter is usually used for children and for laryngectomy patients) and can be uncuffed, cuffed, or fenestrated. The uncuffed tube permits free flow of air around the tube and through the larynx. The plastic cuffed tube provides a low-pressure seal between the trachea and the tube when inflated, allowing for positive-pressure ventilation

EVALUATING COMMON OXYGEN DELIVERY SYSTEMS

Advantages	Disadvantages	Considerations
NASAL CANNULA (Low-flow-system)		
• Comfortable; easily tolerated • Nasal prongs can be shaped to fit facial contour • Effectively delivers low oxygen concentrations • Allows freedom of movement; doesn't impede eating or talking • Inexpensive; disposable	• Contraindicated in complete nasal obstruction, for example, mucosal edema or polyps • May cause headaches or dry mucous membranes if flow rate exceeds 6 liters/minute • Can dislodge easily • Strap may pinch chin if adjusted too tightly • Patient must be alert and cooperative to help keep cannula in place	• Remove and clean cannula every 8 hours with a wet cloth. Give good mouth and nose care. • If patient is restless, explore other methods of oxygen delivery. • Check for reddened areas under nose and over ears. Apply gauze padding, if necessary. • Moisten lips and nose with water-soluble jelly, but avoid occluding the cannula.
SIMPLE FACE MASK (Low-flow system)		
• Effectively delivers high oxygen concentrations	• Hot and confining; may irritate skin • Tight seal necessary to ensure accurate oxygen concentration; may cause discomfort • Interferes with eating and talking • Can't deliver accurate fraction of inspired oxygen (FiO_2) concentration • Impractical for long-term therapy	• Place pads between mask and bony facial parts. • Wash and dry face every 2 hours. • For adequate flush, maintain flow rate of 5 liters/minute. • Remove and clean mask every 8 hours with a wet cloth.
PARTIAL REBREATHER MASK (Low-flow system)		
• Oxygen reservoir bag lets patient rebreathe exhaled air from the trachea and bronchi, increasing FiO_2 concentration • Safety valve allows inhalation of room air if oxygen source fails • Effectively delivers high oxygen concentrations • Easily humidifies oxygen • Doesn't dry mucous membranes • Can be converted to a nonrebreather mask, if necessary	• Hot and confining; may irritate skin • Tight seal necessary to ensure accurate oxygen concentration; may cause discomfort • Interferes with eating and talking • Bag may twist or kink • Impractical for long-term therapy	• Never let bag totally deflate during inhalation. Increase liter flow, if necessary. • Avoid twisting bag. • Keep mask snug to prevent inhalation of room air. • To initially fill bag, apply mask during exhalation.

(continued)

EVALUATING COMMON OXYGEN DELIVERY SYSTEMS *(continued)*

Advantages	Disadvantages	Nursing considerations
NONREBREATHER MASK (Low-flow system)		
• Delivers the highest possible oxygen concentration (60% to 90%) short of intubation and mechanical ventilation • Effective for short-term therapy • Doesn't dry mucous membranes • Can be converted to a partial rebreather mask, if necessary	• Tight seal necessary to ensure accurate oxygen concentration; may cause discomfort • May irritate skin • Impractical for long-term therapy	• Never let bag totally deflate. • Avoid twisting bag. • Keep mask snug to prevent inhalation of room air. • Make sure that all rubber flaps remain in place. • Watch patient closely for signs of oxygen toxicity.
VENTURI MASK (High-flow system)		
• Delivers exact oxygen concentration despite patient's respiratory pattern or if flowmeter knob is bumped • Diluter jets can be changed, or dial-turned, to change oxygen concentration • Doesn't dry mucous membranes • Can be used to deliver humidity or aerosol therapy	• Possibly lowered FIO_2 if air intake ports are blocked • Interferes with eating and talking • Condensation may collect and drain on patient if humidification is being used	• Soften skin around mouth with petrolatum to prevent irritation. • Remove and clean mask every 8 hours with a wet cloth.

and preventing aspiration. Fenestrated tubes have a hole (fenestration) in the outer cannula. This permits speech through the upper airway when the external opening is capped. Many complications are associated with long-term use of tracheostomy tubes (see *Combating complications of tracheostomy*).

Volume-cycled ventilator. This machine is commonly used on a patient who requires long-term ventilation. The volume-cycled ventilator delivers a preset tidal volume under positive pressure, expanding the alveoli and providing better gas exchange. The amount of pressure delivered varies with the patient's lung compliance. The patient is usually sedated, because the natural tendency is to "fight" the uncontrolled ventilation by coughing. The ventilator can regulate virtually every facet of the patient's respiration, including oxygen concentration (21% to 100%), alveolar (or "sigh") distention, tidal volume, end inspiratory pressure, and many others. The main complication associated with ventilator use is infection. Warmth and humidity used in air delivery become conducive to bacterial growth in the system and, subsequently, in the patient's lungs.

COMBATING COMPLICATIONS OF TRACHEOSTOMY

Prevention	Detection	Treatment
ASPIRATION		
• Evaluate patient's ability to swallow. • Elevate his head and inflate cuff during feeding and for 30 minutes afterward.	• Assess for dyspnea, tachypnea, rhonchi, crackles, excessive secretions, and fever.	• Obtain chest X-ray, if ordered. • Suction excessive secretions. • Give antibiotics, if necessary.
BLEEDING AT TRACHEOSTOMY SITE		
• Don't pull on the tracheostomy tube; don't allow ventilator tubing to do so. • If dressing adheres to wound, wet it with normal saline solution and remove gently.	• Check dressing regularly; slight bleeding is normal, especially if patient has a bleeding disorder.	• Keep cuff inflated, except when suctioning, to prevent edema and blood aspiration. Give humidified oxygen. • Document rate and amount of bleeding. Check for prolonged clotting time. • Assist with Gelfoam application or ligation of a small bleeder.
INFECTION AT TRACHEOSTOMY SITE		
• Always use strict aseptic technique. • Thoroughly clean all tubing. • Change nebulizer or humidifier jar and all tubing daily. • Collect sputum and wound drainage specimens for culture.	• Check for purulent, foul-smelling drainage from stoma. • Be alert for other signs of infection: fever, malaise, increased white blood cell count, and local pain.	• Obtain specimens and administer antibiotics. • Inflate tracheostomy cuff, except when suctioning. • Suction the patient frequently, maintaining sterile technique. • Change soiled dressings.
PNEUMOTHORAX		
• Assess for subcutaneous emphysema, which may indicate pneumothorax. Notify doctor if this occurs.	• Auscultate for decreased or absent breath sounds. • Check for tachypnea, pain, and subcutaneous emphysema.	• Obtain chest X-ray to evaluate pneumothorax or chest tube placement. • If ordered, prepare for chest tube insertion.
SUBCUTANEOUS EMPHYSEMA		
• Make sure cuffed tube is patent and properly inflated. • Avoid displacement by securing ties and using lightweight ventilator tubing and swivel valves.	• Most common in mechanically ventilated patients. • Palpate neck for crepitus, listen for escape of air around tube cuff, and check for excessive swelling at wound sites.	• Inflate cuff correctly or use a larger tube. • Suction patient and clean tube to remove any blockage. • Document extent of crepitus.
TRACHEAL MALASIA		
• Avoid excessive cuff pressures. • Avoid suctioning beyond end of tube.	• Dry, hacking cough and blood-streaked sputum when tube is being manipulated.	• Minimize trauma from tube movement. • Keep cuff pressure below 18 mm Hg.

Emergencies

Accidental extubation. This emergency occurs when the tip of a patient's ET tube is accidentally pulled up over the vocal cords and out of the trachea. The cause is usually either faulty anchoring of the tube or deliberate removal by a disoriented patient. Suspect extubation if the ET tube looks abnormally long, if the patient is coughing excessively, or if he's anxious and agitated. In the ventilated patient, the low-pressure and spirometer alarms will sound.

If you suspect your patient may be extubated, notify your instructor or staff nurse. If the cuff is inflated and the tube is above the vocal cords, the tube will slide out easily. The tube will be removed, and temporary airway and respiration established. This involves placement of an oropharangeal plastic airway and ventilation with a bag-valve-mask device.

Acute respiratory failure (ARF), respiratory arrest.
When respiratory arrest occurs without a preceding cardiac event, it's usually the result of ARF, a condition in which $PaO_2 < 50$ mm Hg or $PaCO_2 > 50$ mm Hg. Common postoperative conditions that lead to ARF include pneumonia, pulmonary edema, pulmonary emboli, aspiration, and oversedation. These conditions may cause alveolar hypoventilation, intrapulmonary shunting, ventilation-perfusion mismatch, and decreased diffusion across the respiratory membrane, all of which impair gas exchange. Regardless of the underlying mechanism, ARF implies that the lungs no longer efficiently exchange carbon dioxide for oxygen to keep pace with cellular metabolism.

Diagnostic studies that help confirm diagnosis and etiology of ARF include ABG analysis, chest X-ray, bedside spirometry, sputum gram stain and culture, EKG, and pulmonary artery catheterization.

If ARF progresses to respiratory arrest, the patient stops breathing and subsequently loses consciousness. In the absence of breath sounds, begin pulmonary resuscitation immediately and monitor cardiac status. Follow these steps:
• Open the airway.
• If there's no respiration, call a code.
• Begin mouth-to-mask resuscitation.
• Use an oral airway with a bag-valve mask to ventilate the patient if endotracheal intubation will be delayed.
• Prepare for endotracheal intubation.
• Place the patient on a cardiac monitor.

Pulmonary embolus (PE). A PE occurs when a mass lodges in a branch of the pulmonary artery, obstructing blood flow to the area supplied by the pulmonary vessel. The mass is most commonly a thrombus that forms in the legs or pelvis (deep vein thrombosis) and travels to the lungs via the venous system.

TENSION PNEUMOTHORAX

In tension pneumothorax, air accumulates intrapleurally and can't escape. Intrapleural pressure rises, compressing the ipsilateral lung. The arrows below indicate air movement and pressure within the lung.

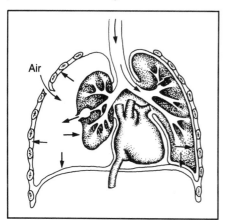

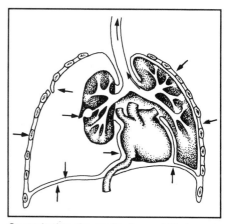

On inspiration, air enters the unaffected lung and the pleural space and becomes trapped.

On expiration, the mediastinum shifts toward the unaffected lung, impairing both ventilation and venous return to the heart.

Prolonged bed rest and immobility promote venous stasis, which can result in thrombus formation.

How PE affects your patient depends on the degree of pulmonary involvement. Signs and symptoms can be subtle or pronounced. In massive PE, the patient will experience sudden onset of dyspnea, anxiety, hypoxia, hypotension, diaphoresis, and decreased organ perfusion. In milder cases, a sudden onset of labored breathing may be the only sign. Patients with suspected PE will probably undergo EKG testing, lung scintigraphy, pulmonary angiography, or magnetic resonance imaging. (For treatment, see the interventions for "Decreased Tissue Perfusion [Pulmonary]," page 84).

Tension pneumothorax. As discussed earlier, this condition develops when a pleural leak, acting as a one-way valve, allows air to accumulate in the pleural space under pressure. In the postoperative patient, the two most common causes of tension pneumothorax are rupture of a bleb (in ventilated patients) and internal leakage from a lung resection. As intrapleural air accumulates, positive pressure builds, causing the trachea, esophagus, heart, and ipsilateral lung to be compressed. The resulting mediastinal shift is the hallmark of tension pneumothorax. On auscultation, you'll hear tracheal sounds to the right or left of the midline (mediastinal shift) on the side opposite the pneumothorax. (See *Tension pneumothorax*). In postoperative patients, air may escape through the suture line, and subcutaneous emphysema may be present.

Signs and symptoms associated with tension pneumothorax include shortness of breath, signs and symptoms of decreased cardiac output (dyspnea, tachycardia, pallor, decreased urine output, and altered level of consciousness), cyanosis, and hypoxemia. Emergency treatment involves immediate decompression of the pleural space (the doctor inserts a large-bore needle to aspirate air) followed by chest tube insertion and establishment of a closed chest drainage system.

Tracheal extubation. If your patient's tracheostomy tube is expelled accidentally, you must take immediate measures to ensure a patent airway. If the tracheostomy is recent, the edges of the skin on either side of the incision will close when the tube is removed, blocking air from entering or escaping through the tracheostomy. Immediately call your instructor or staff nurse, who will use a hemostat, tracheal dilator, or forceps to open the skin folds. This will allow the patient to breathe until help arrives and a new tracheostomy tube is inserted. As a safety measure, an extra tracheostomy tube of the same size and a hemostat should be kept at the bedside.

Upper airway obstruction. This condition involves a blockage of air in the pharynx or trachea. The obstruction may be partial or complete and may result from tumor, vocal cord spasm or paralysis, edema of the epiglottis and larynx, or infections of the pharynx or trachea. Foreign body aspiration is the most common cause of complete airway obstruction in the conscious patient.

Diagnosis of airway obstruction is usually made by clinical observation. Tests to help identify the nature of the obstruction include chest X-rays, soft tissue films of the neck, ABG analysis, pulmonary function studies, and laryngoscopy or bronchoscopy.

When caring for the patient with a possible airway obstruction, ask the patient to speak. If he can speak, his airway is only partially occluded. Note any cyanosis and listen to his breath sounds. Decreased breath sounds, inspiratory or expiratory stridor, and wheezing are common signs of partial obstruction. In complete airway obstruction, the patient lacks airflow from the nose and mouth, and breath sounds are absent. He quickly lapses into unconsciousness.

If your patient has a partial obstruction and can cough forcefully, don't interfere with his attempts to expel the foreign body. Stay with him at all times. Call for assistance and watch for signs of increasingly impaired air exchange. If the patient's condition deteriorates, manage the situation as if it were a complete obstruction. Intervene by initiating techniques recommended by the American Heart Association. As a last resort, cricothyrotomy or percutaneous transtracheal catheter ventilation may be performed by a trained clinician.

☐ Cardiovascular system

Surgical procedures

Balloon valvuloplasty. This procedure is used to dilate stenosed heart valves. If successful, it eliminates the need for surgery in some patients. In a patient with mitral stenosis, a cardiac balloon catheter is passed into the right atrium and a small hole made through the atrial septum into the left atrium. Following the path of blood flow, the catheter is stopped and inflated when the balloon tip enters the mitral valve. Balloon inflation dilates and releases fibrotic valve cusps, resulting in increased patency. Balloon valvuloplasty also is effective in dilating other heart valves. This procedure is done in the cardiac catheterization lab and carries the same preparatory procedures and precautions as for cardiac catheterizaton.

Cardiac surgery. Cardiac surgery may be classified as open-heart or closed-heart. *Open-heart surgery* involves placing a patient on extracorporeal circulation (cardiopulmonary bypass, the heart-lung machine) during the operative procedure. Examples of *open-heart procedures* include coronary artery bypass grafting (CABG), ventricular aneurysm resection, and mitral valve replacement. *Closed-heart procedures,* which do not require cardiopulmonary bypass, include patent ductus arteriosus repair and implantation of automatic cardiac defibrillators. Postoperative patient management is basically the same for both types of procedures, with hemodynamic instability and other complications more common to open-heart surgery. This section presents some nursing diagnoses and interventions associated with preoperative and postoperative phases of cardiac surgery.

Note: As a student, you may or may not have the opportunity to assist with patient care in the immediate perioperative period. This section aims to provide you with an understanding of what occurs during this critical period and to familiarize you with the nurse's role. If allowed to assist, you should confer with your instructor and the patient's staff nurse beforehand to define your role.

Coronary artery bypass graft (CABG) surgery. CABG is a surgical procedure in which blocked coronary arteries are bypassed using saphenous or internal mammary vessel grafts. The number of obstructions bypassed usually range from one to five. During the procedure, the patient must be placed on extracorporeal circulation (a heart-lung machine) because cardiac arrest is induced with I.V. potassium in order to immobilize the heart for surgical manipulation.

Percutaneous transluminal coronary angioplasty (PTCA). This procedure improves coronary blood flow by increasing the

PERCUTANEOUS TRANSLUMINAL CORONARY ANGIOPLASTY

A balloon-tipped catheter (with balloon inflated) rests in a stenosed coronary artery. The close-ups below show catheter placement in the stenotic artery and how balloon inflation widens the vessel lumen.

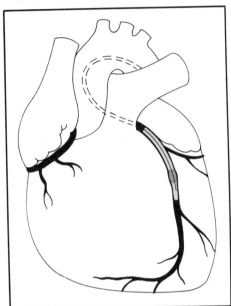

Inflated balloon (dotted line shows catheter entry path)

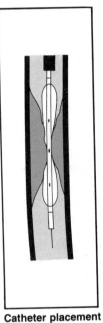

Catheter placement

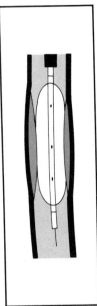

Balloon inflation

lumen size of diseased vessels. A catheter is threaded arterially through the ascending aorta and into the opening of the left coronary artery. A dilating catheter is then inserted through this outer catheter (sheath) using angiography to guide it into the artery's stenosed area. The balloon on the catheter is inflated for 3 to 5 seconds. Angiography is then repeated to evaluate the effect of the procedure. PTCA is a cardiac catheterization procedure that carries the risk of coronary artery occlusion, aortic dissection, myocardial infarction, hemorrhage, and hematoma. Sheaths usually remain in place for 6 to 8 hours after the procedure. Patients usually remain in critical care for observation at least 24 hours. (See *Percutaneous transluminal coronary angioplasty.*)

Valvular surgery. Valvular surgery includes valvuloplasty (valvular repair), annuloplasty (tightening of the valve ring or annulus), commissurotomy (mechanical dilation of the valve), and implantation of a mechanical or bioprosthetic (human or animal) valve. Valvular surgery is an open-heart procedure involving extracorporeal circulation.

Vascular surgery. Vascular surgery is performed to improve circulation to the legs by bypassing diseased vessels. An *aortic bypass* involves anastomosing a Y-shaped synthetic graft above the diseased aortic area (below the renal arteries) and to each femoral artery. A *femoral-popliteal bypass* is most commonly done with a vein harvested from the patient's thigh. *Endarterectomy* or *angioplasty* are two possible alternatives to bypass surgery.

Surgical repair of aneurysms involves clamping the areas above and below the aneurysm, resecting the aneurysm, and anastomosing a synthetic graft in place. (See *Types of vascular repair*, page 96.)

After vascular surgery, patients routinely enter the ICU for 24 to 48 hours for observation. Nursing interventions for these patients focus on assessing pedal pulses, vital signs, and neurologic status.

Preoperative preparation: Vascular surgery

Nursing diagnosis

Knowledge Deficit related to surgical procedure, surgical outcome, and postoperative rehabilitation
Desired outcome: The patient will express an understanding of the procedure and expected course of rehabilitation.

Interventions

1. Assess the patient's level of understanding and discuss the surgical procedure. Be sure to consult with the patient's staff nurse or your instructor before doing so—you may wish to have them present during your initial visit. Use the unit's patient-teaching booklet as a teaching aid.
Rationale: Discussing the patient's surgical concerns reduces his anxiety by increasing his understanding of the procedure and dispelling misconceptions.
2. Have the patient visit the ICU with his family or significant other the day before surgery. With the help of your instructor or the patient's staff nurse, explain the equipment he can expect to see. Explain that he'll be connected to a cardiac monitor and have a nasogastric tube, arterial and central venous pressure (CVP) lines, and an I.V. line inserted. A patient undergoing an aortic bypass may have an abdominal binder as well; tell this patient he must avoid bending his knees and flexing his hips sharply. Provide reassurance and encouragement, but avoid expressing a specific time frame for recovery. Remember that recovery time can vary greatly among patients.
Rationale: Knowing what is going to happen may cause the patient to worry but decreases the immediate postoperative panic and depression often encountered in emergency cases, when

TYPES OF VASCULAR REPAIR

Bypass grafting

Purpose
To bypass an arterial obstruction resulting from arteriosclerosis

Procedure
After exposing the affected artery, the surgeon anastomoses a synthetic or autogenous graft to divert blood flow around the occluded arterial segment. The graft may be synthetic, or it may be a vein harvested from elsewhere in the patient's body.
The illustration at right shows a femoropopliteal bypass.

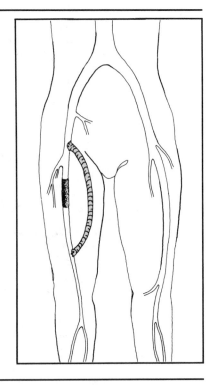

Aortic aneurysm repair

Purpose
To reinforce the wall of the aorta or to remove an aneurysmal segment of the aorta

Procedure
The surgeon first makes an incision to expose the aneurysm site. If necessary, he places the patient on a cardiopulmonary bypass machine; then he clamps the aorta above the aneurysm. Depending on the severity of the aneurysm—and on whether it's ruptured—he wraps the weakened arterial wall with Dacron to reinforce it (shown at right) or replaces the damaged portion with a Dacron graft.

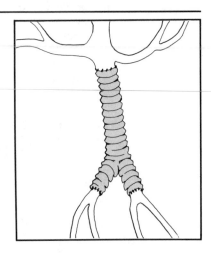

preoperative instruction is not possible. Avoiding discussion of specific time frames for stages of recovery will prevent the patient from comparing himself with others and becoming worried or frustrated at any perceived lack of progress.

Postoperative care: Vascular surgery

See "General postoperative period," page 31, in Section 2.

Nursing diagnosis

Altered Cardiac Output (Decreased): Declining Physiologic and Behavioral Responses related to hypovolemic shock
Desired outcome: The patient will display no signs or symptoms of hypovolemic shock.

Interventions

1. Monitor the patient for:
• hypotension
• tachycardia
• weak or absent peripheral pulses
• pale, cool, clammy skin
• decreased urine output
• tachypnea
• anxiety and restlessness
• complaints of severe back pain (may indicate hemorrhage at the anastomosis site)
• excessive firmness or discoloration of the thighs (may indicate massive blood loss into the thighs)
• decreased hemoglobin and hematocrit
• abdominal distention and absence of bowel sounds (may indicate massive blood loss into the abdomen).
Rationale: These are signs and symptoms of hypovolemic shock.
2. Insert a large-bore I.V. catheter under supervision or, if the patient already has one in place, ensure its patency.
Rationale: A patent I.V. line is required for rapid fluid and drug administration.
3. Administer oxygen by mask or, if indicated, assist trained personnel with intubation.
Rationale: Loss of blood volume results in decreased oxygen transport and eventually tissue hypoxia. Intubation ensures a patent airway for oxygen delivery.
4. Assist with collection of blood samples and monitor the results of laboratory blood tests. These usually include ABG measurements; complete blood count (CBC); electrolyte, blood glucose, blood urea nitrogen (BUN), and creatinine levels; prothrombin time (PT); partial thromboplastin time (PTT); and platelet count.
Rationale: These tests monitor the patient's respiratory and hematologic condition.

Nursing diagnosis

Decreased Tissue Perfusion (Peripheral) related to vascular surgery

Desired outcome: The patient's peripheral perfusion will be maintained.

Interventions

1. As ordered, maintain the patient on bed rest initially, then begin a program of progressive ambulation. Have the patient avoid hip flexion (don't let him sit in a chair, for instance), and elevate the head of the bed no more than 30 to 45 degrees.

Rationale: These precautions will help prevent arterial or graft compression, which can result in decreased blood flow and possibly occlusion.

2. At least every 4 hours, palpate pedal pulses and assess color, temperature, and sensation in the legs, comparing findings for each leg. Mark the location of any pulses that you find difficult to palpate.

Rationale: Changes in findings may indicate graft occlusion.

3. Note and document any areas of discoloration or ecchymosis.

Rationale: Enlarging areas of discoloration or ecchymosis may indicate occult bleeding.

4. For a patient with an aortic bypass, measure and record abdominal girth and auscultate for bowel sounds. Report abdominal distention or absent bowel sounds to the doctor.

Rationale: These findings may indicate hemorrhage at an anastomosis site.

Nursing diagnosis

Ineffective Breathing Pattern related to operative discomfort or prolonged bed rest

Desired outcome: The patient will verbalize pain relief and will exhibit normal bilateral breath sounds and chest excursion.

Interventions

1. Position the patient for optimal comfort, and assist him with repositioning at least every 2 hours.

Rationale: Repositioning allows aeration of all lobes.

2. Administer pain medications, as ordered.

Rationale: Relief of pain allows the patient to deep-breathe more effectively, ensuring aeration of all lung fields.

Nursing diagnosis

Knowledge Deficit related to activities associated with vascular postoperative rehabilitation

Desired outcome: Before leaving the hospital, the patient will verbalize his plan for rehabilitation at home.

Interventions

Teach the patient about permitted activities and his planned progression from one level of activity to another. If a standardized

rehabilitation form is not available on your unit or from the surgeon, ask a nurse or your instructor to help you locate this information. Points to cover generally include:
• incision care
• signs and symptoms of infection (redness, swelling, pain, and increased drainage)
• leg and foot care, including avoiding temperature extremes, leg crossing, and restrictive clothing; exercising as ordered; and wearing antiembolism stockings as ordered
• the need for follow-up examinations.
Rationale: Patient compliance with rehabilitation guidelines enhances recovery.

Preoperative preparation: Cardiac surgery

Nursing diagnosis
Knowledge Deficit related to surgical procedure, surgical outcome, and postsurgical rehabilitation
Desired outcome: The patient will verbalize understanding of the surgical procedure and expected postsurgical rehabilitation.

Interventions
1. Assess the patient's level of understanding and discuss the scheduled surgical procedure. Be sure to consult with the patient's staff nurse before doing so—you may wish to have an experienced nurse or your instructor present during your first visit. Use the unit's patient-teaching booklet as a guide when explaining your patient's specific surgery to him.
Rationale: Anxiety often impairs comprehension. Discussing the patient's surgical concerns reduces his anxiety by increasing his understanding of the procedure and dispelling misconceptions. Preoperative teaching may have to be repeated more than once.
2. Have the patient visit the postoperative recovery room with his family or significant other the day before surgery. With the help of your instructor or the patient's staff nurse, explain the equipment he can expect to see. Explain that he will awaken with an ET tube connected to a ventilator and will not be able to talk; encourage him to plan on using another means of communication, such as writing notes. Also explain that he'll be connected to a cardiac monitor and have a nasogastric tube, chest tubes, epicardial pacing wires, an arterial line, and a pulmonary artery catheter inserted. Point out that, barring complications, the ET tube, ventilator, nasogastric tube, and other equipment may be removed within 16 hours after surgery. However, avoid expressing a specific time frame for recovery to the patient.
Rationale: Knowing what is going to happen may cause the patient to worry but decreases the immediate postoperative panic and depression frequently encountered in emergency cases,

when preoperative instruction is not possible. Avoiding discussion of specific stages of recovery using time frames will prevent the patient from comparing himself with others. Recovery time varies among individual patients. A patient who has been told that "chest tubes come out on the third day" may think something is wrong when his are still in place on the fourth day after surgery.

Postoperative care (immediate): Cardiac surgery

See "General postoperative period," page 31, in Section 2.

Nursing diagnosis

Altered Cardiac Output (Decreased): Declining Physiologic and Behavioral Responses related to cardiogenic shock (shock from pump failure)
Desired outcome: The patient will display no signs or symptoms of cardiogenic shock.

Interventions

1. Monitor the patient for:
• hypotension and narrowing pulse pressure
• tachycardia or bradycardia
• an S_3 heart sound
• weak or absent peripheral pulses
• pale, cool, clammy skin
• decreased urine output
• distended neck veins
• pulmonary congestion
• peripheral edema
• tachypnea
• anxiety and restlessness.
Rationale: These are signs and symptoms of cardiogenic shock, caused by inadequate cardiac output resulting from myocardial damage.
2. Monitor cardiac activity for dysrhythmias and abnormal EKG changes, and report any abnormalities.
Rationale: A damaged, overdistended myocardium is irritable and tends to develop ectopic foci and cause dysrhythmias.
3. Insert a large-bore I.V. catheter under supervision or, if the patient already has one in place, make sure it is patent.
Rationale: A patent I.V. line is necessary for rapid fluid and drug administration.
4. Administer oxygen by mask or, if indicated, assist trained personnel with intubation.
Rationale: A damaged, hypoxic myocardium has increased oxygen demands. Intubation ensures a patent airway for oxygen delivery.

5. Obtain a standard 12-lead EKG and chest X-ray, according to your unit's standing orders or at the doctor's request.
Rationale: A baseline EKG should be obtained as soon as signs and symptoms of pump failure develop. Chest X-ray will reveal the presence and extent of lung congestion and establish heart size.
6. Administer pain medication, as ordered.
Rationale: The patient may have severe ischemic myocardial pain. Administering morphine I.V., as ordered, will relieve pain and also cause peripheral vasodilation, leading to reduced afterload.
7. Under supervision, assist with insertion of an arterial line and pulmonary artery catheter with a thermistor and CVP port for cardiac output readings. In cardiogenic shock, CVP will rise (unless the patient is hypovolemic), pulmonary artery and capillary wedge pressure will increase, and cardiac output will decrease.
Rationale: Cardiac output, pulmonary capillary wedge pressure, and direct, continuous mean blood pressure readings are essential in the management of this disorder. The aim of collaborative therapy is to interpret these readings and therapeutically alter preload and afterload to increase cardiac output.
8. Assist with collection of blood samples and evaluate results of all laboratory tests. These usually include ABG values; CBC; electrolyte, blood glucose, BUN, and creatinine levels; PT; PTT; platelet count; and cardiac enzymes (CK-MB, LDH).
Rationale: These tests indicate the patient's respiratory, hematologic, and myocardial condition.

Nursing diagnosis
Decreased Tissue Perfusion: Cardiac Dysrhythmias related to cardiac irritability secondary to ischemia
Desired outcome: The patient will exhibit no dysrhythmias, or any dysrhythmias that do occur will be identified and controlled with medication.

Interventions
1. Initiate cardiac monitoring, with assistance, and set alarm parameters as instructed.
Rationale: Routine pulse checks alone are inadequate to identify and treat dysrhythmias; cardiac monitoring is necessary.
2. Treat life-threatening dysrhythmias according to standing orders.
Rationale: As a student, you will not actually administer medications, but you can assist the staff nurse by preparing them. Routine standing orders are established in these situations because no time is available to call a doctor for orders.
3. Report frequent ectopy (nonsinus beats, especially those originating in the ventricles) to your instructor, the staff nurse, or the doctor.

Rationale: Ectopy indicates myocardial irritability. Ectopic beats can originate in the atria, nodal-junctional tissue, and the ventricles. Premature ventricular contractions (PVCs) are the most common and the most dangerous. Generally, in postoperative patients, more than eight PVCs per minute, multifocal PVCs (occurring in different sites in the ventricle), and PVCs occurring in couplets or runs (two or more together) should be reported and treated promptly.

Nursing diagnosis
Ineffective Breathing Pattern related to pain or discomfort from chest tubes
Desired outcome: The patient will verbalize pain relief and will exhibit normal bilateral breath sounds and chest excursion.

Interventions
1. Position the patient for optimal comfort, and assist him with repositioning at least every 2 hours.
Rationale: Repositioning allows aeration of all lobes.
2. Administer pain medications, as ordered.
Rationale: Relief of pain allows the patient to deep-breathe more effectively, ensuring aeration of all lung fields.

Nursing diagnosis
Impaired Gas Exchange related to bronchial secretions and shallow breathing
Desired outcome: The patient's ABG values and breath sounds will remain within normal limits.

Interventions
1. Monitor ABG values from the patient's chart.
Rationale: ABG values provide the most definitive indication of ventilatory status. Normal values: $pH = 7.35$ to 7.45, $PaO_2 = 80$ to 100 mm Hg, and $PaCO_2 = 35$ to 45 mm Hg.
2. Have the patient turn, cough, and deep-breathe (TCDB) every 2 hours; assess breath sounds.
Rationale: TCDB helps expel bronchial secretions that clog airways and prevent gas exchange. Frequent evaluation of breath sounds helps assess aeration and congestion.

Postoperative cardiac rehabilitation

Nursing diagnosis
Knowledge Deficit related to activities associated with postoperative rehabilitation
Desired outcome: Before leaving the hospital, the patient will verbalize his plan for rehabilitation at home.

Interventions
1. Teach the patient the principles of exercise tolerance and initial cardiac recovery. Explain the relationship between overexer-

tion, increased myocardial oxygen demand, and myocardial ischemia. Regardless of the specific recovery regimen, instruct the patient to immediately stop any activity that results in chest pain, palpitations, shortness of breath, or a pulse rate of 25 beats or more above his resting rate.

Rationale: A patient's understanding of the relationship between increased activity and myocardial ischemia usually leads to increased compliance and effectiveness of rehabilitation.

2. Teach the patient about permitted activities and his planned progression from one level of activity to another. If a standardized rehabilitation form is not available on your unit, ask a nurse or your instructor to help you locate this information.

Rationale: Most patients are anxious about being discharged from the hospital and have very specific questions, usually related to allowed activities—particularly sexual intercourse.

3. Make sure the patient has written guidelines for any special diet that is ordered.

Rationale: The patient may not remember or understand certain aspects of his diet and may need a repeat dietary consultation before discharge.

4. Have the patient, his family, or his significant other explain his medication regimen to demonstrate understanding. Discharge medication instructions should include the dosage amount and schedule, possible adverse reactions, and precautions for each prescribed drug.

Rationale: Most postoperative patients are discharged with an extensive medication regimen. They are concerned about such things as adverse reactions, drug incompatibilities, and instructions for missed doses. These fears aren't without foundation; many of these medications (digoxin and warfarin, for example) can be dangerous if not taken as ordered.

Nursing diagnosis

Knowledge Deficit related to bacterial endocarditis prophylaxis
Desired outcome: The patient will relate an understanding of disease process and state prophylactic measures for prevention of bacteremia.

Interventions

1. Explain the disease process and the need for long-term antibiotic therapy.

Rationale: A patient with existing cardiac lesions or a prosthetic valve is prone to reinfection.

2. Discuss the need for special antibiotic prophylaxis prior to invasive procedures. A patient scheduled to undergo dental, genitourinary, gynecologic, or GI procedures should inform the dentist or doctor of his cardiac condition beforehand.

Rationale: Bacteria may be introduced into the bloodstream during invasive procedures. Abnormal turbulent blood flow through affected heart valves encourages bacterial vegetative growth in the valve area.

3. Teach the patient to watch for and promptly report early indicators of infection, including elevated temperature, malaise, and flulike symptoms.

Rationale: Early detection and treatment with appropriate antibiotics improve the course of recovery.

Diagnostic tests

Angiography, coronary (cardiac catheterization). This test assesses coronary artery blockage or occlusion that may result in myocardial tissue damage (vascular insufficiency) and determines the extent of the restricted blood flow. The procedure may also be used to deliver streptokinase to occluded areas in an attempt to dissolve blood clots and clear blockages.

In this procedure, a catheter is inserted into an artery in the antecubital fossa or into the femoral artery and guided under fluoroscopy in a retrograde fashion through the aorta to the openings of the coronary arteries (where the aorta meets the left ventricle). A contrast medium is then injected into the coronary artery opening and X-rays made of the medium's progress through the vessels. Fluoroscopic filming of the heart's activity can provide information on mitral and aortic valve function, left ventricular function, and coronary artery patency.

Blood pool imaging, first-pass and gated. Cardiac blood pool imaging is performed to evaluate ventricular function, to detect myocardial wall abnormalities, and to detect intracardiac shunting. In *first-pass imaging,* a radioisotope (technetium 99m) is injected, then a scanner records the radioactivity emitted by the isotope in its initial pass through the heart. The function of each heart chamber can be evaluated as the isotope makes its way from the superior vena cava into the right atrium, right ventricle, pulmonary system, left atrium, left ventricle, and on out through the aorta. The heart is imaged only during cardiac cycles in progress during the first pass of the isotope; after these initial cycles, presence of the isotope within all heart chambers and systemic dilution prohibit further evaluation. First-pass imaging is useful in assessing cardiac function both at rest and after exercise.

In *gated imaging,* or *multiple gated acquisition (MUGA) scanning,* a camera records ventricular end systole and end diastole for 500 to 1,000 cardiac cycles following an injection of isotope-tagged red blood cells (RBCs). Computerized superimposition of these images enables evaluation of left ventricular function.

MUGA scanning can be performed at rest or while exercising to assess ventricular function.

Chest X-ray. A chest X-ray usually is ordered to determine the size, shape, and placement of the heart. Routine evaluation involves posteroanterior and left lateral views. For a posteroanterior chest X-ray, the patient stands on the floor and rests his chin on top of an X-ray cassette holder in front of him. He is asked to take a deep breath and hold it for the duration of the X-ray (a few seconds), and the film is exposed. For the left lateral view, the patient is positioned with his arms over his head and his torso against the film cassette. The procedure is painless and requires only the patient's cooperation.

Digital subtraction angiography (DSA). This procedure enhances standard contrast angiography with computer processing to produce high-resolution images of cardiovascular structures. It accomplishes this by digitally subtracting extraneous structures, such as bone and soft tissue, that may interfere with visualization of the desired structure. Although this procedure is used primarily for carotid and renal studies, its applications in cardiology include evaluation of coronary arterial flow, myocardial perfusion, and left ventricular function.

Doppler ultrasonography. This noninvasive ultrasound procedure is used to evaluate blood flow in veins and arteries. A hand-held transducer directs high-frequency sound waves to the artery or vein being tested. The sound waves strike moving RBCs and are reflected back to the transducer at frequencies that correspond with the velocity of blood flow through the vessel (the higher the frequency, the higher the velocity). The transducer then amplifies the sound waves to allow direct listening or graphic recording.

Echocardiography (M-mode, two-dimensional, and color). This noninvasive test uses ultrahigh-frequency sound waves to evaluate the size, shape, and motion of cardiac structures. This procedure enables assessment of myocardial thickness and movement; overall left ventricular function; mitral valve prolapse; mitral, tricuspid, and pulmonic insufficiency; cardiac tamponade; pericardial diseases; cardiac tumors; prosthetic valve function; subvalvular stenosis; ventricular aneurysms; cardiomyopathies; and congenital abnormalities.

Electrocardiography (resting, standard, and multichannel EKG). A resting EKG is ordered to detect myocardial infarction, myocardial ischemia, conduction problems, dysrhythmias, or chamber enlargement, or to assess the effects of electrolyte imbalance or cardiac medications. A total of 12 electrodes placed on the patient's limbs and chest wall receive electrical impulses generated by depolarization and repolarization of the heart. The electrodes are connected by lead wires to the EKG machine, which converts the incoming electrical signals into a graphic display. Each electrode represents a "channel", and electrical activity is recorded from the direction of each electrode position, resulting in 12 different electrical views of the heart. A standard EKG records one channel at a time; a multichannel EKG records three consecutive leads simultaneously.

EKG, ambulatory (Holter monitoring). A continuous ambulatory EKG is used to detect sporadic dysrhythmias that may be missed by exercise or resting EKGs. It is particularly helpful in detecting dysrhythmias in patients who complain of intermittent cardiac symptoms but show no evidence of dysrhythmias on a resting EKG and in uncovering myocardial electrical instability after myocardial infarction. It also can be used to monitor the effects of medications on the heart or can be tailored to other patient needs and research applications. The patient usually wears five electrodes connected to a small, battery-operated EKG recorder secured to a waist-belt. The recorders available for patient use vary, but most are capable of two-channel (simultaneous two-lead) monitoring. For a period of 24 hours, the device continuously records the patient's heart rate as the patient keeps a written record (diary) of his activities—such as walking, stair climbing, sleeping, and sexual activity. In addition, when the patient feels a cardiac symptom, such as chest pain, palpitations, or any unusual sensation, he presses an event button on the EKG recorder to mark the onset of symptoms on the Holter EKG paper. Later, on analysis, this mark and the subsequent EKG tracing are correlated with the patient's diary. Some ambulatory monitoring recorders are patient-activated (intermittent) and do not run continuously for 24 hours. Instead, the patient wears the monitor for 5 to 30 days and presses the event button to record only those instances when he feels symptoms.

EKG, exercise (stress test). An exercise EKG enables evaluation of cardiac activity during periods of physical stress. Unlike a resting EKG, this test monitors electrical activity while the heart's demand for oxygen is increased by exercise. The procedure is commonly used to evaluate chest pain and to determine the functional capacity of the heart after myocardial infarction. It also enables screening of patients for asymptomatic coronary artery disease and dysrhythmias on exertion and monitoring of the effectiveness of cardiac medications. This procedure is usually conducted by a doctor, with the assistance of a nurse or technician. The patient is connected to a blood pressure gauge and EKG monitor while exercising on a treadmill or stationary bicycle ergometer. Both blood pressure and cardiac activity are monitored while the patient exercises toward a predetermined target heart rate or until he develops fatigue or chest pain. Many stress-testing systems are programmed to automatically increase cardiac work load and record periodic EKGs during the procedure.

Technetium pyrophosphate scanning (hot-spot imaging). This procedure detects recent myocardial infarction and determines the extent of damage. It is especially useful in patients complaining of obscure cardiac pain and patients whose EKGs are not diagnostically definitive. In this procedure, technetium 99m pyrophosphate is injected into the bloodstream through the antecubital vein. The tracer isotope accumulates in damaged myocardial tissue, where it forms a "hot spot" on a nuclear scan made with a scintillation camera. Hot spots can appear within 12 hours of infarction but are most apparent 48 to 72 hours postinfarction.

Thallium scanning (cold-spot imaging). This test is performed to evaluate myocardial blood flow and the status of myocardial damage postinfarction. It also is used to diagnose coronary artery disease (stress imaging) and to evaluate bypass graft patency, antianginal therapy, or balloon angioplasty. The procedure involves an I.V. injection containing thallium 201, which concentrates in healthy myocardial tissue but not in necrotic or ischemic tissue. Areas of poor blood flow and damaged tissue fail to take up the isotope and appear as "cold spots" on a nuclear scan. This procedure is effective within the first few hours postinfarction but cannot differentiate an old infarct from a new infarct. The scan can be done with the patient resting or after exercising on a treadmill. In exercise thallium scanning, stress-induced ischemia can be detected as increased cold spotting.

Equipment, tubes, and drains

Arterial lines. An arterial line is used in patient assessment to evaluate systolic, diastolic, and mean arterial pressures and to calculate systemic vascular resistance in the most accurate, rapid, and comfortable manner. Other uses for the arterial line include obtaining blood samples for ABG analyses and other frequently performed laboratory tests. This eliminates a significant amount of patient discomfort. An arterial line usually is a 20G Teflon over-the-needle catheter that has been placed in an artery, attached to tubing and a transducer, and connected to a monitor that displays arterial waveforms on an oscilloscope. The artery used depends on the sites that are safe and readily available in each patient. Arteries commonly used are the radial, brachial, femoral, and dorsalis pedis. The radial artery is used most often because of the collateral circulation provided by the ulnar and palmar arteries. This reduces the risk of permanent injury from arterial cannulation by having alternate routes of blood supply available should an occlusive problem arise in the radial artery. The brachial artery may be used if the radial artery is not available.

Cardiac monitors. A patient is placed on a cardiac monitor to observe for and detect dysrhythmias and other abnormalities in cardiac conduction and function. Alarms can be set to alert the nurse to rate problems, and printouts of cardiac rhythms can be documented at the bedside or central station, depending on the sophistication of the monitoring system. The electrodes are placed on the chest wall in a lead II, MCL, or lead I position. The lead that shows the best QRS waveform is usually chosen for continuous cardiac monitoring. Electrodes pick up electrical impulses from muscles of the heart and chest wall, and an attached cable transmits them to a monitor that displays the impulses as waveforms on an oscilloscope.

Chest tubes (mediastinal tubes) and closed chest drainage. See "Chest tubes, closed drainage systems," page 85.

Pulmonary artery catheter. The pulmonary artery or Swan-Ganz catheter is a balloon-tipped flow-directed catheter used to indirectly measure left heart pressure. The catheter may be inserted into the internal jugular, subclavian, or, in some cases, antecubital vein. The balloon end floats the catheter into the right atrium, through the tricuspid valve, and into the pulmonary artery. During diastole, pulmonary artery pressure reflects left ventricular end diastolic, or left heart, pressure. Inflation of the catheter's balloon tip in the pulmonary artery blocks out right heart pressure. Left heart pressure is picked up by the catheter and transducer, then transmitted to an oscilloscope for display as pressure waves. In addition to left heart pressure, more sophisticated catheters can be used to measure CVP and cardiac output and to perform as a pacing wire.

Emergencies

The American Heart Association designates two types of emergency life-support procedures: basic life support (BLS) and advanced cardiac life support (ACLS). All nursing students must pass BLS in order to qualify for clinical experience through the various hospital rotations.

As a student nurse, you will not be expected to participate in a resuscitation. However, you can help the code team by understanding the steps involved in ACLS and anticipating their needs. If you find a nonresponsive patient or if a patient goes into cardiac arrest while you are caring for him, you need to know what to do in those first few minutes and what to do after a code team arrives.

If you witness a cardiac arrest and your patient becomes unresponsive, take the following steps:
1. Make sure the patient is unresponsive.
2. Open the airway and "look, listen, and feel" for respiration.

3. If the patient is not breathing, ALERT THE RESUSCITATION TEAM. (Call a code.)

4. Place the patient on a firm surface. Most of the newer hospital beds provide adequate rigidity. If you're not sure, use a cardiac board or a food tray. Do not delay the start of cardiopulmonary resuscitation (CPR) looking around for a board. In minutes, you will have assistance and other personnel can locate it. Do not place the patient on the floor, unless his collapse makes this unavoidable—certain procedures, such as femoral or subclavian I.V. insertion, are difficult when the patient is on the floor. Also, more people can have simultaneous access to the patient if he is in bed.

5. Begin CPR and do not stop until relieved by another certified CPR practitioner. CPR should be maintained by members of the code team until a perfusable rhythm is obtained or the code is discontinued by a doctor.

6. If you have practiced this procedure, attach monitor or defibrillator electrodes to the patient in a lead II pattern. Simultaneously, the team may use "quick look" paddles that pick up an EKG tracing when applied to the chest. (*Note:* The paddles will not function as electrodes on some defibrillators if the patient cable remains connected to the machine.) If the patient is in ventricular fibrillation or ventricular tachycardia (with no pulse), someone from the team may decide to defibrillate him immediately.

7. Prepare the materials to start an I.V. (5% dextrose in water; administration set; 14G, 16G, and 18G catheters; and an I.V. tray). You will not be expected to cannulate a vessel during an arrest. Usually, the doctor will place the I.V. in the femoral or subclavian vein once the code is underway.

8. Prepare for intubation and oxygenation. A respiratory therapist is probably part of your code team. Don't count on team members being there immediately; they may be at another emergency. If you know what the doctor will need, you can help. The person managing the respiratory part of resuscitation will need an oxygen flowmeter, tubing, Ambu bag, laryngoscope with straight and curved adult blades, an assortment of ET tubes sizes 7 to 10, an ET tube obturator, tape, and an ET tube adapter. A suction source with tubing attached to a Yankauer catheter or large-bore suction catheter should be on hand. In the event that the patient regurgitates stomach contents, it may be necessary to use the blunt end of the suction tubing to clear the mouth. If possible, find these items on the crash cart and practice working with them before a code occurs (for example, connecting the blade to the laryngoscope).

9. Document events and monitor vital signs.

10. Support the family; remove them from the scene of the arrest.

11. Remove other patients from the scene of the arrest.

12. Anticipate and obtain necessary items from the crash cart and floor stock.

Steps in airway management:

1. Opening the airway and ensuring its patency.

2. Giving mouth-to-mouth resuscitation (mouth-to-mask resuscitation is recommended by the Centers for Disease Control).

3. Inserting an oral airway and ventilating with a bag-valve mask while awaiting intubation.

4. Performing endotracheal intubation and positive-pressure breathing.

Steps involved in chest compression, including adjuncts for artificial circulation:

1. BLS chest compression; one-person and two-person CPR.

2. Automatic chest compression. An automatic chest compressor is used most often by emergency personnel in the field to resuscitate victims in situations where not enough rescuers are available to do BLS and ACLS or when transporting a patient in areas where CPR is impossible (such as down a flight of stairs). In the hospital, it may be used if a long resuscitation is anticipated or if the rescuers become fatigued. The machine is powered by compressed oxygen, and most models can provide synchronized ventilation as well as chest compression.

Steps in monitoring and defibrillation:

If you have practiced beforehand, you can confidently apply the electrodes and obtain an EKG reading on the oscilloscope while waiting for the team. If you are familiar with the defibrillator, you can set the wattage and charge the unit under supervision, when instructed to do so.

Other tips:

1. Learn the dysrhythmias associated with cardiac arrest. This knowledge will enable you to anticipate which medications will be used, and in what order.

2. Be familiar with the defibrillation procedure—especially those steps that will ensure your safety and the safety of those around you.

☐ Gastrointestinal (GI) system

Surgical procedures

Abdominal herniorrhaphy. This procedure surgically repairs herniation (or protrusion) of the intestine though a weakened area of the abdominal wall, returning the intestine to the abdominal cavity. Emergency herniorrhaphy may be indicated when intestinal strangulation could lead to ischemia and eventually gangrene. Hernioplasty involves reinforcing the weakened area with mesh or wire.

Antireflux surgery and hiatal hernia. A hiatal hernia is a stomach pouch that has passed through the esophageal hiatus into the chest. The chief complaints of patients with hiatal hernia are "heartburn" (gastric reflux) and associated chest pain. This disorder is usually controlled by adjusting the patient's diet and administering antacids and other medications. As a last resort, antireflux surgery is considered. (See *Antireflux surgery*, page 112, for a description of this procedure.)

Appendectomy. This procedure is done to remove an inflamed appendix, preferably prior to rupture (perforation) with resulting peritonitis. Routine preoperative education is required, and prophylactic antibiotics may be ordered. Routine postoperative turning, coughing, deep breathing, pain medication administration, and ambulation also are required. The patient may or may not have a nasogastric (NG) tube and abdominal drains in place; clarify this with the surgeon (see "Preoperative period" and "Postoperative period" in Section 2.).

Gastric procedures for ulcer disease. The chart below describes common surgeries to treat ulcer disease. Names of gastric surgeries (other than vagotomy) commonly refer to the stomach portion removed. Most procedures combine two surgeries. (See *Gastric surgeries for ulcer disease,* pages 114 and 115.) *Note:* Keep in mind that "-ostomy" means "an opening into." If only one prefix precedes "-ostomy," then the surgical opening is made from the exterior—for example, gastrostomy. Two prefixes indicate anastomosis—for example, gastroenterostomy (anastomosis of a stomach [gastro-] remnant with a small intestinal [-entero-] segment).

Ileostomy procedures. The patient with inflammatory bowel disease may require an *ileostomy*—creation of a stoma from the ileum for waste elimination. An ileostomy usually accompanies total colon and rectum removal. Waste (liquid or semisolid, as the patient no longer has a colon to absorb water) then flows through the stoma virtually constantly. An ostomy appliance fitted over the stoma collects the waste and prevents it from flowing onto the skin, where it can cause irritation. Special skin-care and odor-control measures must be taken to ensure patient comfort.

Some patients with ulcerative colitis now have an alternative to conventional ileostomy: the continent Kock pouch or the ileal pouch-anal anastomosis. The *continent Kock pouch* involves construction of an intra-abdominal reservoir, or pouch, with a nipple valve from the patient's terminal ileum. The pouch is then

ANTIREFLUX SURGERY

All three surgical procedures for reflux esophagitis leave at least part of the stomach surrounding the lower esophagus.

The illustration at right shows Hill's repair, in which the surgeon sutures the posterior phrenicoesophageal ligament to the median arcuate ligament. He wraps the fundus around the terminal esophagus.

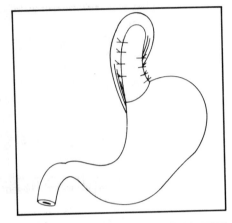

In Belsey's repair, illustrated at right, traction on the sutures invaginates the esophagus into the stomach. This repair can be done above or below the diaphragm.

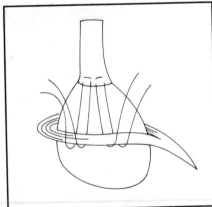

The illustration at right shows Nissen's repair, which wraps the stomach's fundus around the terminal esophagus and sutures it there.

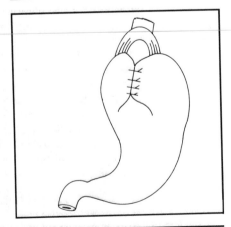

sutured to the abdominal wall. Ileostomy discharge is stored in the pouch until the patient drains it using a catheter. No appliance is required. An *ileal pouch–anal anastomosis* permits removal of the colon and rectum with a permanent ileostomy. The procedure preserves the anal sphincters and preserves voluntary anal defecation and fecal continence.

Ostomy procedures. The patient with intestinal cancer or another intestinal disorder, such as bowel injury, fistula, chronic diverticulitis, or chronic inflammatory disease, may need a *colostomy*—formation of an outside abdominal opening (stoma) from a section of colon. A colostomy may be *permanent*, if the patient requires removal of a large section of the intestine, including the rectum and anus, or *temporary*, if the patient has a diseased, inflamed, or injured bowel that requires rest. As shown on the chart below, colostomies take their names from the surgical site: *ascending, transverse, descending,* or *sigmoid* (see *Types of colostomies,* page 116).

Preoperative preparation

Nursing diagnosis

Potential for Infection related to inadequate bowel preparation
Desired outcome: The patient will not develop a postoperative abdominal infection.

Interventions

1. Strictly adhere to bowel preparation prescribed by the doctor.
Rationale: Bowel preparations are aimed at clearing fecal matter and eliminating bacteria from the bowel. An incomplete preparation could result in a serious postoperative infection.
2. Administer a low-residue diet or give nothing by mouth, as directed.
Rationale: Even the presence of clear liquids in the bowel can contribute to postoperative infection.
3. Report any problems with bowel preparation to the patient's doctor.
Rationale: Surgical bowel preparation is a major factor in avoiding postsurgical infection. Surgery may be cancelled if desired effects are not obtained.
4. Document findings accurately and completely.
Rationale: An accurate description of bowel preparation results should be included in the patient's permanent record.

Nursing diagnosis

Knowledge Deficit related to surgical procedure and postoperative events
Desired outcome: The patient will verbalize an understanding of the surgical procedure and postoperative events.

GASTRIC SURGERIES FOR ULCER DISEASE

Type	Effects	Indications
VAGOTOMY		
Truncal (total abdominal vagotomy)	• Cuts vagus nerve at esophageal base • Destroys vagal innervation of stomach and abdomen • Destroys gastric, intestinal, and gallbladder motility • Stops acid production	• Recurrent ulcer disease (usually combined with pyloroplasty) • Acid reduction
Selective	• Cuts vagus nerve • Destroys vagal innervation of stomach (but retains abdominal innervation) • Stops acid production	• Recurrent ulcer disease (usually combined with pyloroplasty) • Acid reduction
Highly selective (parietal cell vagotomy)	• Cuts parietal cell branches of vagus nerve • Denervates acid-producing cells but doesn't affect motility	• Recurrent ulcer disease • Acid reduction
PYLOROPLASTY		
	• Enlarges pylorus by removing sphincter effect in pyloric channel • Gives stomach and duodenum free communication	• Pyloric stricture or obstruction (may be combined with vagotomy)
GASTRECTOMY		
Billroth I (B-I) (gastroduodenostomy, hemigastrectomy)	• Resects antrum and anastomoses gastric remnant to proximal duodenum • Destroys antral function and pyloric sphincter • May cause bile reflux	• Gastric ulcer • Pyloric obstruction

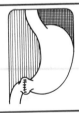
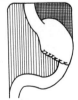

GASTRIC SURGERIES FOR ULCER DISEASE *(continued)*

GASTRECTOMY (continued)

Type	Effects	Indications
Billroth II (B-II) (gastrojejunostomy) 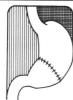	• Resects antrum and anastomoses gastric remnant to proximal jejunum (retains duodenum) • Destroys antral function • Allows digestive secretions of liver and pancreas to mix in duodenum • Duodenum serves as afferent loop; proximal jejunum, as efferent loop	• Duodenal ulcer • Pyloric obstruction
Total gastrectomy (esophagojejunostomy)	• Resects stomach from lower esophageal sphincter to duodenal bulb; anastomoses duodenum and esophagus • Destroys gastric function; ingested materials pass from esophagus to duodenum	• Ulcer disease • Pyloric obstruction • Gastric cancer
Gastric resection (antrectomy)	• Removes stomach portion • Effects depend on portion removed (for example, antrectomy alters digestive function)	• Recurrent ulcer disease • Perforation

Interventions

1. Explain the surgical procedure to the patient after the doctor has done so.

Rationale: The patient may not have understood the doctor's explanation or may have misconceptions about surgery or unrealistic expectations regarding the outcome.

2. Have patient demonstrate breathing and splinting exercises and leg exercises.

Rationale: Postoperative pain and anxiety tend to decrease compliance with planned therapy. Preoperative practice facilitates postoperative compliance.

3. Explain GI decompression using an NG tube or a Salem sump tube.

Rationale: Patients may have NG or other intestinal tubes inserted preoperatively or postoperatively. The GI tube and suction equipment are frightening to the patient if he is not aware of their purpose.

TYPES OF COLOSTOMIES

Type		Features
ASCENDING COLON		
Ascending colostomy	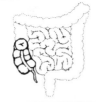	• Requires full-time use of odor-proof, drainable pouch and skin barrier to protect skin from corrosive digestive enzymes • Produces discharge that usually appears watery or semisolid and may be continuous
TRANSVERSE COLON		
Single-barrel colostomy		• Frequently temporary • Requires full-time use of odor-proof, drainable pouch and skin barrier to protect skin from corrosive digestive enzymes • Produces discharge that usually appears pastelike or semisolid and may occur frequently and at unpredictable intervals
Double-barrel colostomy	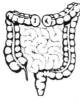	
Loop colostomy		
DESCENDING OR SIGMOID COLON		
Descending colostomy	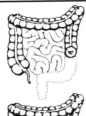	• Sometimes called "dry" colostomy because colon may still produce formed stools, although patient lacks voluntary control • May require irrigation (an enema administered through stoma) daily or every other day and may regulate discharge enough to prevent unpredictable bowel movements (irrigate stoma according to doctor's orders) • No pouch necessary if dependable irrigation pattern can be established. Single-use closed stoma pouch or disposable security pouch required otherwise
Sigmoid colostomy	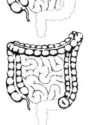	

4. Discuss anticipated postoperative incisional tubes and drains. *Rationale:* Knowing what to expect decreases postoperative anxiety. A patient unaware of the routine use of wound drains, for example, may think his condition has worsened upon finding them if they are not described as routine beforehand. When the patient sees serosanguineous drainage, he may think he's hemorrhaging.
5. Have the patient make a preoperative visit to the ICU if he is scheduled to return there postoperatively. *Rationale:* Such equipment as a cardiac monitor, for example, is not expected by the patient and may cause him to think he has developed heart problems. Take an experienced nurse along if the patient wishes to make the preoperative visit to ensure that all his questions are answered.

Postoperative care

Nursing diagnosis
Altered Tissue Perfusion (Multisystem): Decreased Physiologic and Behavioral Responses related to hemorrhagic shock
Desired outcome: The patient will experience no signs and symptoms of hypovolemic shock.

Interventions
1. Check incision for bright-red bleeding.
Rationale: Cause of shock could be massive wound hemorrhage, evidenced by leakage through incision.
2. Check volume of wound drainage in suction apparatus (Hemovac).
Rationale: A large volume of bright-red blood is an indication of wound hemorrhage.
3. Monitor vital signs every 15 minutes if shock is suspected.
Rationale: Patients in shock have a blood pressure (BP) less than 90/60 and are tachycardic.
4. Observe for coolness of extremities, decreased level of consciousness, decreased CVP, and decreased urine output.
Rationale: These signs further confirm the diagnosis of shock.
5. Place patient in Trendelenburg's position if shock is suspected.
Rationale: This position facilitates venous return to vital organs.
6. Check patency and size of I.V. catheter. Prepare to administer dextrose 5% in lactated Ringer's solution at a rate sufficient to raise systolic BP to 90 mm Hg.
Rationale: I.V. catheter should be at least 16G or 18G to accommodate the increased flow of I.V. fluid, blood, and plasma expanders given throughout resuscitation.
7. Have the crash cart readily accessible.
Rationale: If the patient loses consciousness, he will need to have a patent airway established and be ventilated, as required.

Nursing diagnosis

Altered Bowel Elimination: Absence of Stool related to paralytic ileus

Desired outcome: The patient's peristaltic bowel function will return to normal within 2 days after surgery.

Interventions

1. Auscultate for bowel sounds 1 full minute in each quadrant.
Rationale: Bowel sounds may be faint or occur infrequently as they return. They should return within 2 days after surgery.
2. Ask the patient whether he is passing flatus or stool.
Rationale: Passage of flatus or stool indicates the return of peristalsis.
3. Keep the patient mobile. Ambulate if not contraindicated at least four times a day.
Rationale: Mobility helps restore peristalsis.
4. Measure abdominal girth if abdomen becomes distended.
Rationale: Distention should be monitored because it can place tension on the suture line or indicate other problems, such as hemorrhage or ascites.
5. Ensure patency of NG tubes and any other GI tubes in place. Irrigate with normal saline solution, when ordered (to prevent additional electrolyte losses).
Rationale: Tube obstruction can result in accumulation of gas and secretions.
6. Resume a progressive diet (clear liquids to solid food) slowly as bowel sounds return.
Rationale: The patient cannot tolerate a regular diet immediately after resumption of peristalsis.
7. Insert a rectal tube, if allowed.
Rationale: Insertion of a rectal tube helps eliminate gaseous distention of the sigmoid colon.

Nursing diagnosis

Altered Comfort: Pain related to abdominal incision

Desired outcome: The patient will verbalize relief or control of pain.

Interventions

1. Administer pain medications 20 minutes before dressing changes or intensive coughing and deep-breathing sessions.
Rationale: This allows time for analgesic and sedative actions of the medications to take effect.
2. Instruct the patient to splint his abdomen with a pillow while coughing.
Rationale: This maneuver helps control pain by decreasing movement of abdominal muscles.

Nursing diagnosis

Potential for Infection: Abdominal Rigidity and Tenderness related to peritonitis
Desired outcome: The patient will not develop peritonitis.

Interventions

1. Monitor vital signs for elevated temperature and tachycardia.
Rationale: These signs correlate with other findings in the diagnosis of peritonitis.
2. Assess abdomen for rigidity and tenderness.
Rationale: These are "peritoneal signs" that indicate irritation of the abdominal cavity.
3. Check bowel sounds every 30 minutes if peritonitis is suspected.
Rationale: Paralytic ileus usually accompanies peritonitis; bowel sounds will be diminished or absent.
4. Monitor hematology profile.
Rationale: Elevated white blood cell (WBC) count usually accompanies the evolution of peritonitis.
5. Document findings.
Rationale: These findings should be included in the patient's permanent preoperative record.

Diagnostic tests

Abdominal CT scan. This test uses a computer to translate the action of multiple X-ray beams into three-dimensional oscilloscopic images that help identify abscesses, cysts, hematomas, tumors, and pseudocysts. In addition, it is used to evaluate pancreatic and biliary disorders. The test can be performed with or without contrast dye.

Abdominal flat plate. This X-ray study helps evaluate and detect tumors, kidney stones, abnormal gas collection, obstruction, and other abdominal disorders. The test consists of two X-rays, one taken with the patient supine and the other with the patient upright.

Endoscopy. This procedure involves direct visualization of the GI tract using an endoscope. Glass fibers inside the flexible tube-shaped endoscope transmit light and return an image of the GI lumen, permitting visualization of inflammation, bleeding, neoplasms, or any other lesions. Biopsy specimens can also be obtained by attaching forceps. Endoscopic examinations include colonoscopy, gastroscopy, and proctosigmoidoscopy.

Hematologic tests. Selected blood tests for GI disorders include alkaline phosphatase, ammonia, amylase, bilirubin, cholesterol, gamma glutamyl transpeptidase, lactic dehydrogenase, lipase, prothrombin time, and transaminases.

Nuclear imaging. This study analyzes concentrations of injected or ingested radiopaque substances. Gastric emptying studies use radionuclides to evaluate the ability of the stomach to empty solids or liquids in emptying disorders. Liver-spleen scanning is used to detect hepatocellular disease and hepatic metastatic lesions.

Ultrasonography. In this technique, sound waves emitted from an ultrasound probe create echos that appear as an image on an oscilloscope. This study can diagnose biliary disorders, abdominal tumors, abscesses, and hematomas.

Equipment, tubes, and drains

Abdominal drains. After abdominal surgery, the patient may need an abdominal drain to remove secretions while his wound heals. The type of drain used depends on the wound's size and location as well as the type and expected amount of drainage. Various abdominal drains are illustrated and described in the chart on the opposite page.

Esophageal tubes. An esophageal tube is inserted by the doctor to help control or stop esophageal bleeding. These tubes, such as the Sengstaken-Blakemore, Linton-Nachlas, and Minnesota tubes, have inflatable balloons (esophageal, gastric, or both) that compress esophageal blood vessels and provide pressure over bleeding sites. However, they also may cause such complications as airway obstruction, esophageal edema, ulceration, and necrosis.

Intestinal tubes. When caring for a patient with an intestinal obstruction, you may need to help place an intestinal tube and provide continuing care. These tubes (such as the Miller-Abbott, Cantor, and Harris tubes), used for diagnostic or physiologic studies, most commonly serve to decompress the small bowel.

Nasogastric (NG) tubes. The purpose of an NG tube is to establish a route for administration or removal of fluid (or air) to and from the stomach. There are various types of NG tubes, each slightly different and designed for a specific gastric problem. The chart on page 123 reviews NG tubes, their features, and indications for use.

Emergencies

Evisceration. Evisceration refers to the extrusion of abdominal organs (viscera) as a result of trauma or failure of sutures in a surgical incision. If this occurs, immediately cover the exposed viscera with sterile, normal saline solution–soaked pads. *Note: Do not attempt to push the viscera back into the abdominal cavity!*

ABDOMINAL DRAINS

Penrose drain

The most common abdominal drain, this flat, short, single-lumen tube works through capillary action. Used for uncomplicated draining wounds of moderate size, it won't damage surrounding tissue or cause serious inflammation.

Cigarette drain

Simply a Penrose drain stuffed with gauze, this drain also suits uncomplicated draining wounds of moderate size. The gauze helps draw up fluid, augmenting the drain's capillary action.

Two-in-one drain

Another variation of the Penrose, this contains fenestrated tubing, which also increases capillary action. The tubing can be connected to suction if necessary.

Sump drain

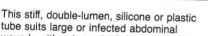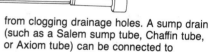

This stiff, double-lumen, silicone or plastic tube suits large or infected abdominal wounds with substantial fluid output. The outer lumen has several openings for air entry, which helps keep adjacent tissues from clogging drainage holes. A sump drain (such as a Salem sump tube, Chaffin tube, or Axiom tube) can be connected to constant low-pressure suction.

Triple-lumen sump drain

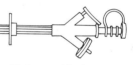

This drain (for example, an Abramson tube) performs three functions—irrigation, suction, and passage of filtered air over the wound. Medication or irrigating solution can be removed by continuous suction. The doctor will choose this drain for large or infected complicated abdominal wounds, especially those contaminated through perforation or trauma.

T tube

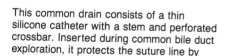

This common drain consists of a thin silicone catheter with a stem and perforated crossbar. Inserted during common bile duct exploration, it protects the suture line by diverting about a third of the 1,000 ml of bile secreted daily by the liver. It can also remove small stones from the bile ducts.

(continued)

ABDOMINAL DRAINS *(continued)*

Indwelling catheter

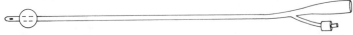

Ordinarily used to drain the bladder, this catheter can also serve as a drainage device for the stomach or gallbladder. (Inflating the balloon on a Foley catheter reduces the risk of the drain falling out.) Malecot (batwing) and dePezzer (mushroom) catheters also serve this purpose.

Closed-suction drain

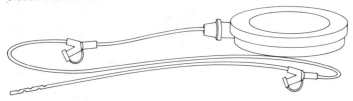

This self-contained system—a collapsible device attached to a flat, narrow drain with multiple openings—exerts negative pressure to withdraw accumulated fluids. Systems such as Reliavac, Hemovac, J-VAC, and the Jackson-Pratt device (the latter shaped differently than shown) can be used to drain a wide, flat area with little tissue displacement. The doctor may also use such a system when he anticipates large drainage amounts or when lesser amounts may delay healing.

Notify the doctor immediately and assess the patient for signs and symptoms of shock. Stay with the patient and provide emotional support until he is sent to surgery for wound closure.

GI bleeding. Common causes of upper GI bleeding include gastritis, peptic ulcer, and esophageal varices. Less common causes include Mallory-Weiss syndrome (mucosal lining tear associated with forceful vomiting) and Boerhaave's syndrome (esophageal perforation associated with bulimia). Emergency interventions in GI bleeding usually include:
• insertion of an esophageal tamponade balloon (Sengstaken-Blakemore tube) for bleeding esophageal varices
• administration of crystalloid (such as Ringer's lactate) or colloid (such as albumin) solution through a large-bore I.V. catheter
• administration of RBCs
• gastric lavage with iced normal saline solution through a large-bore NG tube
• drug therapy (vasoconstrictors, norepinephrine, antacids, histamine blockers)
• endoscopic injection sclerotherapy (injection of a coagulating substance into a bleeding varix).

Peritonitis. A thin, shiny, continuous membrane, the peritoneum lines the abdominal cavity. The parietal peritoneum lines the ab-

NASOGASTRIC TUBES

Tube	Features	Indications
Levin	• Single lumen; 42" to 50" (107 to 127 cm); rubber or plastic with holes at tip and along side	• Aspiration of gastric contents (including fluid and gas) • Gastric lavage • Drug administration • Enteral feeding • Diagnostic studies
Salem-Sump	• Double lumen; 48" (122 cm); clear plastic with blue sump port (pigtail); openings at sides and tip; markings at 45, 55, 65, and 75 cm • Radiopaque line • Air vent lumen (pigtail port) allows atmospheric air to enter patient's stomach so tube can float freely, preventing tube from adhering to and damaging gastric mucosa. Larger port serves as main suction tube	• Aspiration of gastric contents (including fluid and gas) • Gastric lavage • Drug administration • Enteral feeding • Diagnostic studies (*Note:* Always keep blue pigtail above level of patient's stomach to prevent reflux of gastric contents into vent lumen. Use large lumen to irrigate tube. After irrigation, instill air into pigtail lumen.)
Moss	• Triple lumen; #20 French tube • Radiopaque tip • First lumen, positioned and inflated at cardia, serves as balloon inflation port; second lumen, as esophagogastric aspiration port; third lumen, as duodenal feeding port	• Aspiration of gastric contents after surgery (tube placed intraoperatively) • Prevention of postoperative ileus • Duodenal feeding within 24 hours postoperatively
Ewald	• Single lumen; large bore with several openings at distal end • Allows large fluid volumes to enter and leave stomach quickly	• Gastric lavage of blood or after poison ingestion or drug overdose • Short-term use (removed after lavage and evacuation of stomach contents)
Levacuator	• Double lumen; large bore • Large lumen allows for evacuation of stomach contents; small lumen permits irrigant instillation	• Gastric lavage of blood or after poison ingestion or drug overdose • Short-term use (removed after lavage and evacuation of stomach contents)
Edlich	• Single lumen; large bore with four openings near closed distal tip	• Gastric lavage of blood or after poison ingestion or drug overdose • Short-term use (removed after lavage and evacuation of stomach contents)

dominal wall and the visceral peritoneum covers the abdominal organs. Between the parietal and visceral layers lies the peritoneal cavity.

By secreting a serous lubricating fluid, the peritoneum functions mainly to provide a frictionless surface, permitting free abdominal visceral movement. The peritoneal surface also acts as a membrane for the selective passage of water and solutes in both directions across the membrane.

Peritonitis—peritoneal inflammation—may occur when a perforated abdominal organ (such as the bowel or gallbladder) leaks fluid and blood into the abdominal cavity, causing infection or irritation. Peritonitis may be primary or secondary, acute or chronic.

Signs and symptoms depend on the site and extent of inflammation and may include abdominal pain, abdominal rigidity, nausea, vomiting, increased temperature, and tachycardia. Treatment includes:
• identifying the cause
• promoting fluid and electrolyte balance
• controlling pain
• providing gastric or intestinal decompression.

PERITONEAL TAP AND LAVAGE

Peritoneal tap (paracentesis) and lavage help detect intraabdominal bleeding. To perform a *peritoneal tap* (shown in the top illustration, below left), the doctor introduces a catheter or trocar into the patient's peritoneal cavity (see the close-up, below right). (The tap may be done in one or more abdominal quadrants; however, most doctors now do a single tap just superior to the umbilicus.) Gross blood, bile, urine, or fecal matter apparent on peritoneal cavity puncture indicates bleeding, which warrants surgery.

If no gross blood or other material appears initially, the doctor may then perform *peritoneal lavage* (shown in the bottom illustration, below left). This involves rapid infusion of 1 liter of fluid (usually normal saline solution or Ringer's lactate solution) into the peritoneal cavity. The patient may be gently rolled from side to side (unless he has skeletal injuries) or tilted slightly (if his vital signs permit) so fluid can reach all intraabdominal areas and mix with any blood. (In some cases, the patient's abdomen may be manipulated manually instead.) Fluid is then collected by gravity drainage into a collection container placed lower than the abdomen. A positive lavage shows return of bloody, pinkish-red fluid, dark enough to obscure newsprint held behind the drain tubing. If the newsprint is readable, the doctor will probably consider the lavage negative, although he may order further diagnostic tests. Fluid sample analysis includes complete blood count, amylase, bile, culture, and Gram stain.

Other abnormal findings include green (bile-stained) fluid, which may indicate bowel perforation; cloudy or turbid fluid, a possible sign of bowel infarction or peritonitis from bowel rupture; and milky (chyle-containing) fluid, which suggests small intestine perforation. (Normal peritoneal fluid appears clear to pale yellow.)

Keep these points in mind if the doctor has ordered peritoneal tap or lavage for your patient:
• If ordered, assist with nasogastric tube insertion before the procedure to decompress the stomach.
• Have the patient void before the procedure, or insert an indwelling (Foley) catheter, as ordered.

Trauma. Abdominal trauma and internal bleeding are difficult to evaluate because of referred pain and the presence of many overlapping organs. Peritoneal lavage is a common diagnostic test administered when internal hemorrhage is suspected. (See *Peritoneal tap and lavage.*)

In addition, the *Guide to abdominal trauma*, pages 127 and 128, will assist you in reviewing specific organ injuries and their management.

☐ Biliary system and pancreas

Surgical procedures

Biliary surgery includes cholecystectomy (removal of the gallbladder), cholecystostomy (opening of the gallbladder to remove gallstones), and choledochostomy (opening of the common bile duct for stone removal), as well as procedures for placement of hepatic catheters and portacaval shunts. Two procedures for gallstone removal are outlined in *Removing retained gallstones: Two techniques,* page 130. Pancreatectomy involves removal of all or part of the pancreas. (See *Whipple procedure [Pancreatoduodenectomy],* page 131.)

• Maintain a sterile field and strict sterile technique during the procedure.
• To allow fluid to flow back into the container, make sure the I.V. tubing doesn't have a non-backflow filter. If you're using an I.V. bottle setup, break off the air vent's plastic tubing so a water seal doesn't form.
• Apply an antibiotic ointment and sterile dressing after catheter or trocar removal.
• After the procedure, observe for complications, such as bowel or bladder perforation and free air in the peritoneal cavity.

Peritoneal tap

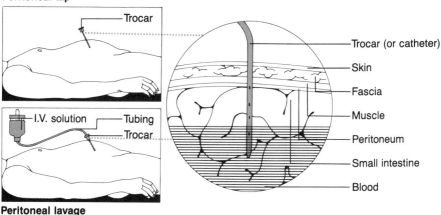

Trocar

I.V. solution — Tubing
Trocar

Peritoneal lavage

Trocar (or catheter)
Skin
Fascia
Muscle
Peritoneum
Small intestine
Blood

Preoperative preparation

Nursing diagnosis

Altered Comfort: Pain related to bile obstruction from gallstones or gallbladder spasms

Desired outcome: The patient will verbalize relief of pain or state that pain has lessened.

Interventions

1. Administer pain medications as needed.

Rationale: The patient may have intermittent attacks of pain preoperatively.

2. Tell the patient to report intense pain not relieved within 30 minutes after taking medications.

Rationale: This may indicate acute bile duct obstruction, which may necessitate surgery.

Nursing diagnosis

Potential for Injury: Abdominal Tenderness and Rigidity related to chemical irritation of the peritoneum by bile (chemical peritonitis)

Desired outcome: If chemical peritonitis occurs, the nurse will rapidly identify and report it.

Interventions

1. If the patient complains of abdominal pain or discomfort, assess for abdominal rigidity and pain on palpation.

Rationale: These signs and symptoms are associated with peritonitis.

2. Monitor vital signs closely.

Rationale: Elevated temperature correlates with other findings in the assessment of peritonitis.

3. Monitor hematologic profile.

Rationale: WBC level usually is elevated in peritonitis.

Nursing diagnosis

Knowledge Deficit related to surgical procedure and postoperative events

Desired outcome: The patient will verbalize an understanding of the surgical procedure and postoperative events.

Interventions

1. Explain the surgical procedure to the patient after the doctor has done so.

Rationale: The patient may not have understood the doctor's explanation or may have misconceptions about the procedure or unrealistic expectations regarding its outcome.

2. If the patient is scheduled to receive a T tube, explain the device and how it helps bile drainage.

Rationale: A patient who does not understand the purpose of surgical tubes and drains may become anxious when such a de-

GUIDE TO ABDOMINAL TRAUMA

Liver	Spleen	Pancreas	Stomach and small intestine
POSSIBLE CAUSES			
Blunt or penetrating trauma to upper right or left quadrants, epigastric area (as from steering wheel injury, high-impact motor vehicle accident, or fall), or both	Blunt or penetrating trauma (as from fall, high-impact motor vehicle accident, or direct impact resulting from contact sports)	Blunt trauma to epigastric area (as from fistfight, steering wheel injury, or bicycle handlebar impact)	*Stomach*—usually penetrating trauma (as from stab or gunshot) *Small intestine*—usually blunt trauma (as from kick or seat-belt injury)
ASSESSMENT			
History of trauma to right or left quadrants, epigastric area, or both; upper quadrant pain, tenderness, or rigidity; possibly referred pain to shoulder	History of trauma to left upper quadrant, left upper quadrant pain and rigidity, Kehr's sign (referred pain to left shoulder)	History of blunt epigastric trauma, ecchymosis in epigastric region, nonspecific abdominal signs and symptoms (pain may occur immediately, decrease over the next 2 hours, then increase again)	History of upper abdominal trauma *Stomach*—upper abdominal pain, decreased bowel sounds, evidence of peritoneal irritation *Small intestine*—nonspecific abdominal signs and symptoms (may not appear until 12 to 18 hours after injury), ecchymosis in epigastric region, absent bowel sounds
SPECIFIC DIAGNOSTIC TESTS			
Computed tomography (CT) scan, peritoneal tap or lavage	CT scan, arteriography, peritoneal tap or lavage	CT scan, serum amylase (elevated)	Upright abdominal X-ray (may show air), alkaline phosphatase (elevated), CT scan, contrast upper GI series
INTERVENTIONS			
• Ensure airway, breathing, and circulation (ABCs). • Intervene for hypovolemic shock, if indicated. • Prepare for surgery, if indicated. • Enforce bed rest and observe closely if patient doesn't undergo surgery.	• Ensure ABCs. • Intervene for hypovolemic shock, if indicated. • Prepare for surgery, if indicated.	• Ensure ABCs. • Intervene for hypovolemic shock, if indicated. • Prepare for surgery, if indicated. • Administer treatment for pancreatitis, if indicated.	• Ensure ABCs. • Intervene for hypovolemic shock, if indicated. • Prepare for surgery, if indicated. • Administer broad-spectrum antibiotics, as ordered. • Decompress stomach.

(continued)

GUIDE TO ABDOMINAL TRAUMA *(continued)*

Colon and rectum	Kidneys and ureters	Bladder and urethra	Vasculature
POSSIBLE CAUSES			
Colon—penetrating trauma to lower abdomen (as from stab or gunshot) *Rectum*—penetrating trauma (as from foreign body)	*Kidneys*—blunt trauma (as from motor vehicle accident, direct impact, or fall) *Ureters*—penetrating trauma	Blunt trauma to lower abdomen (as from direct impact or falling astride object)	Blunt or penetrating trauma
ASSESSMENT			
History of penetrating trauma to lower abdomen, subcutaneous emphysema, absent bowel sounds	History of trauma to area, hematuria, costovertebral angle or flank pain, tenderness or rigidity, oliguria or anuria, local ecchymosis	History of trauma to area; lower abdominal or suprapubic pain; inability to void despite stronge urge, or hematuria; ecchymosis on lower abdomen or perineum	History of blunt or penetrating trauma, abdominal tenderness or rigidity, evidence of hypovolemic shock (retroperitoneal hemorrhage may not produce signs and symptoms of shock), Cullen's or Turner's sign
SPECIFIC DIAGNOSTIC TESTS			
Colon—peritoneal tap or lavage (positive for blood or bacteria) *Rectum*—gross blood	I.V. pyelogram, renal arteriogram	Pelvic X-rays, cystogram or urethrogram, I.V. pyelogram	Arteriogram
INTERVENTIONS			
• Ensure ABCs. • Intervene for hypovolemic shock, if indicated. • Prepare for surgery, if indicated. • Administer broad-spectrum antibiotics, as ordered, to reduce sepsis risk.	• Ensure ABCs. • Intervene for hypovolemic shock, if indicated. • Prepare for surgery, if indicated. • Enforce bed rest and observe closely if patient doesn't undergo surgery.	• Ensure ABCs. • Intervene for hypovolemic shock, if indicated. • Prepare for surgery, if indicated. • *Don't* catheterize if you note bleeding at urinary meatus (doctor may insert suprapubic catheter). • Enforce bed rest and administer analgesics and sitz baths if patient doesn't undergo surgery.	• Ensure ABCs. • Intervene for hypovolemic shock (use medical antishock trousers, if necessary). • Prepare for surgery. • *Don't* start I.V. in the patient's leg because fluid may escape into abdominal cavity.

vice is inserted and may possibly misinterpret insertion as a sign that his condition is worsening.
3. Explain the principles of gastric decompression and the need for I.V. therapy during this procedure.
Rationale: Postoperatively, a patient becomes thirsty from dry mouth and prolonged mouth breathing. However, drinking is not permitted during gastric decompression. I.V. fluid therapy compensates for the lack of oral intake. Suggest that the patient use lemon-glycerin swabs (and ice chips, if permitted) to relieve dry mouth.
4. Tell the patient to expect to receive no food by mouth for up to 3 days postoperatively, and explain that I.V. fluids will provide the necessary nutrients during this period.
Rationale: The patient should know what to expect during the immediate postoperative period.
5. Explain the expected extent of surgery to a patient scheduled to undergo pancreatectomy.
Rationale: Patients should have realistic expectations about the outcome of their surgery. Removal of the pancreas is major, extensive surgery that also may involve removal of adjacent organs. Check with the doctor for anticipated postsurgical prognosis.

Postoperative care

Nursing diagnosis
Altered Comfort: Pain related to surgical incision
Desired outcome: The patient will verbalize that pain has been controlled or relieved.

Interventions
1. Administer prescribed pain medication 20 minutes before major dressing changes and intensive coughing and deep-breathing sessions.
Rationale: Incisions for biliary and pancreatic surgery are made high on the abdominal wall, making coughing and deep breathing painful for many patients.
2. Apply an abdominal support (binder) over the incision site.
Rationale: This will help the patient sit up and move more comfortably.
3. Teach the patient to splint his abdomen with a pillow while coughing and deep breathing.
Rationale: This will support abdominal muscles by decreasing movement and associated pain.

Nursing diagnosis
Impaired Skin Integrity related to irritating drainage from Penrose drain
Desired outcome: The patient's skin will remain intact with no erythema.

REMOVING RETAINED GALLSTONES: TWO TECHNIQUES

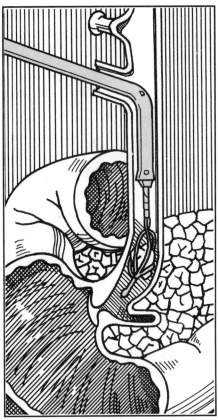

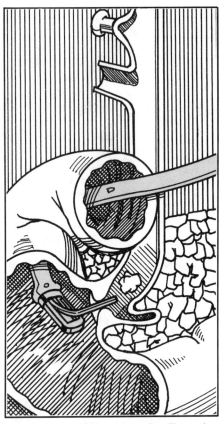

The doctor can remove retained stones by snaring them with a Dormia basket. He introduces the basket through a choledochoscope or catheter in the T-tube tract.

In endoscopic sphincterotomy (papillotomy), the doctor removes the retained stones with a Dormia basket or Fogarty catheter. By cutting the papilla or the sphincter of Oddi, he creates a larger opening into the duodenum, allowing other retained stones (or future stones) to pass into the duodenum.

Interventions

1. Change dressings whenever you note drainage or at least once a day, as ordered.

Rationale: Frequent dressing changes prevents prolonged contact of irritating drainage with skin.

2. Apply a waterproof skin protectant, such as petrolatum, Karaya, or zinc oxide, around the incision and drain.

Rationale: This repels drainage and helps protect skin.

3. If copious drainage necessitates more than two dressing changes every 8 hours, apply a closed ostomy bag over the drain.

WHIPPLE PROCEDURE (PANCREATODUODENECTOMY)

In this technique, the doctor resects the stomach, duodenum, pancreas, and bile duct. He may also remove the gallbladder. Three anastomoses connect the common bile duct, pancreas, and stomach to the jejunum. The doctor anastomoses the pancreas and bile duct proximal to the gastric anastomoses to neutralize acidic secretions dumped from the stomach into the jejunum. He may also perform a vagotomy to decrease gastric acid secretion.

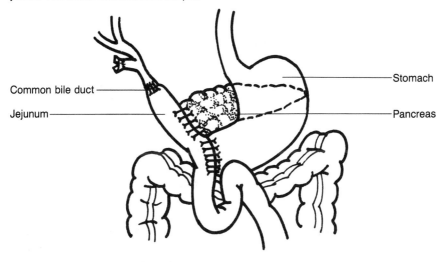

Common bile duct

Jejunum

Stomach

Pancreas

Rationale: An ostomy bag collects drainage and keeps it from contacting the skin.

Nursing diagnosis

Potential for Injury: Jaundice related to blocked bile duct or T tube

Desired outcome: The nurse will identify jaundice early and report it immediately.

Interventions

1. Assess the patient for yellowed sclera and skin and dark-brown urine.

Rationale: These are signs of jaundice, a common preoperative and postoperative complication of biliary surgery.

2. Ensure T-tube patency.

Rationale: A blocked T tube prevents bile drainage, possibly resulting in postoperative jaundice.

3. Monitor and record T-tube drainage every shift.

Rationale: As edema in the common bile duct subsides, the amount of T-tube drainage should decrease gradually. A sudden decrease may indicate blockage.

Nursing diagnosis

Potential for Infection: Abdominal Pain and Tenderness related to subhepatic abscess secondary to intraoperative liver damage
Desired outcome: The patient will not develop subhepatic abscess.

Interventions

1. Assess for swelling and complaints of pain and tenderness over the liver and throughout the entire right upper abdominal quadrant, possibly radiating to the right shoulder and back. Report persistent or increasing pain not relieved by pain medications.
Rationale: Such pain is a common symptom of subhepatic abscess.
2. Monitor vital signs closely.
Rationale: Fever and tachycardia often accompany subhepatic abscess.
3. Teach the patient to report any flulike symptoms and malaise.
Rationale: Such symptoms may indicate infection.

Diagnostic tests

Angiography. This test is used to detect small, early-stage pancreatic tumors before they can be detected by CT scan or ultrasonography.

Cholescintigraphy. In this study, technetium 99m–labeled hepatobiliary agents are injected I.V., and a gamma camera takes serial images over an hour to record the agents' progress through the liver, bile ducts, gallbladder, and duodenum. This test can pinpoint obstructed areas, but it lacks the resolution to detect stones.

CT scans. CT scanning can help evaluate pancreatic size, shape, and density using a contrast study.

Endoscopic retrograde cholangiopancreatography (ERCP). ERCP uses both radiography and endoscopy to examine the pancreatic ducts and hepatobiliary tree. In this procedure, the doctor advances a small side-viewing endoscope through the patient's mouth, esophagus, stomach, and duodenum until he identifies the ampulla of Vater. He then injects a contrast medium by passing a cannula through the endoscope.

ERCP helps diagnose suspected pancreatic and biliary duct disease. It is also used to locate cysts, calculi, and stenosis in the pancreatic ducts and hepatobiliary tree, particularly when other radiographic studies, such as ultrasonography, CT scans, liver scans, and biliary tract X-rays, yield inconclusive findings.

I.V. cholangiography. In this radiologic study, the biliary system is visualized through a series of X-rays taken over several

T-TUBE CARE: SOME TIPS

Nursing measure	Benefit
Avoid kinking of or tension on tube by securing tube to patient's gown with pin or tape.	Prevents flow obstruction and avoids tension on suture site.
Place drainage bag at abdominal level.	Prevents excessive bile loss by allowing flow when biliary tree pressure increases.
Observe and record drainage amount, color, and any unusual conditions (for example, odor).	Helps detect complications, such as obstructions, fistulas, clots, leakage, or dislodgement.
After clamping (as ordered), check for and record such signs and symptoms as pain, nausea, vomiting, bloating, and chills.	Assesses patient tolerance—an index of bile flow adequacy.
Monitor fluid, electrolyte, and acid-base status; report drainage amounts exceeding 500 ml in a 24-hour period.	Prevents fluid, electrolyte, and acid-base imbalance (excess bile loss can lead to metabolic alkalosis).
Return bile, as necessary, by replacing it orally or through nasogastric tube (best given chilled in fruit juice).	Aids fat digestion.
Protect patient's skin from bile drainage.	Prevents skin excoriation from exposure to bile.

hours after dye is injected I.V. Ducts should be visible within 30 minutes, the gallbladder within 4 hours. *Note:* This test is rarely performed because of the high rate of allergic reactions.

Oral cholecystography. This is a radiologic study that visualizes the gallbladder and the bile duct system using an oral iodine-based dye. The liver extracts the dye from the blood and releases it into the bile. If the gallbladder does not visualize on X-ray, an obstruction of the gallbladder or duct system (by spasm or stones) is suspected.

Percutaneous transhepatic cholangiography (PTC). This test involves injection of radiopaque dye directly into the liver biliary tracts using a needle inserted through the eighth or ninth intercostal space. PTC differentiates hepatic from extrahepatic jaundice and detects stricture, stenosis, and obstructions by tumors or stones.

Ultrasonography. This procedure has largely replaced cholecystography and now is the primary noninvasive test for patients with jaundice. The test involves "scanning" the upper abdomen with an ultrasonic probe, which produces an image of the abdominal viscera and enables visualization of gallstones or thickening of the gallbladder. Ultrasonography also is used to detect pancreatic enlargement, neoplasms, calcification, cysts, abscesses, and fibrous infiltrate.

TRANSHEPATIC BILIARY CATHETER: CARE TIPS

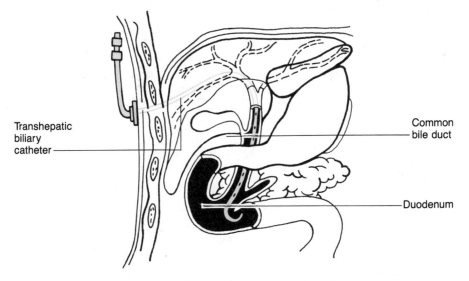

Transhepatic biliary catheter

Common bile duct

Duodenum

The doctor may insert a transhepatic biliary catheter—an internal bile drain—as a palliative therapy when nonresectable liver, pancreatic, or biliary duct cancer obstructs bile flow. This measure may also relieve signs and symptoms of biliary obstruction and hepatic dysfunction secondary to obstructive jaundice or biliary sepsis. Although not a cure, the procedure permits a more normal life-style.

The doctor inserts the catheter fluoroscopically through the abdominal wall, liver, and common bile duct, passing through or by the obstruction to the duodenum. Holes in the catheter allow bile to drain into the duodenum, preventing it from accumulating in the liver.

Before the procedure, explain to the patient that catheter insertion may take several hours and cause pain. Because this procedure punctures the liver, the patient should have laboratory studies the day before to rule out bleeding disorders. If needed, fresh frozen plasma will be ordered. Withhold food and fluids the day of the procedure. The doctor will order pain medication and possibly antibiotics.

After catheter insertion, monitor vital signs frequently for indications of hemorrhage and sepsis. An external drainage bag, attached for several days, allows ductal edema to subside. Observe drainage for quantity,

color, odor, and consistency. Report excessively bloody drainage immediately—this may indicate catheter dislodgment in a hepatic blood vessel. If drainage exceeds 1,500 ml in 24 hours, suspect retrograde duodenal content flow, an intestinal obstruction, or both.

Irrigate the catheter with a syringe containing 5 to 20 ml of sterile saline solution, as ordered. Use of a three-way stopcock, with the drainage bag attached, eases irrigation. Once edema subsides, and if the patient shows no complications, the drainage bag is removed and the catheter capped, as ordered, to allow bile to drain into the duodenum. With the bag removed, irrigation takes place through the external port. Don't force the irrigant against resistance, and don't aspirate it. If the patient develops cramping or pain, notify the doctor.

Keep the insertion site clean and dry. Report any bile leakage around the catheter.

Assess the patient for signs of adequate catheter function, such as resolving jaundice and normal urine and stool color.

Before discharge, teach the patient and his family how to irrigate and care for the catheter. Also teach him which signs and symptoms of malfunctions or complications to report. Consider home health care referrals, if needed.

Equipment, tubes, and drains

T tubes. This T-shaped tube is usually inserted after exploration of the common bile duct. The tube permits bile drainage during healing despite swelling and inflammation of the bile duct postoperatively. See *T-tube care: Some tips*, page 133, for guidelines on caring for a patient with a T tube in place.

Transhepatic biliary catheter. This internal bile drain is used in palliative therapy for patients with nonresectable biliary, pancreatic, or hepatic cancer. It relieves symptoms associated with obstruction of bile by bypassing the obstruction to the duodenum. For a description of the procedure and information on catheter care, see *Transhepatic biliary catheter: Care tips*.

Emergencies

The most common emergency is rupture of the gallbladder with subsequent development of peritonitis. Rupture often is preceded by jaundice. This represents a medical emergency requiring immediate notification of the doctor. (See "Peritonitis," page 122.)

☐ Musculoskeletal system

Surgical procedures

Surgery for the musculoskeletal system is performed to treat pain and immobilization. Procedures include amputation, open reduction and internal fixation, laminectomy and spinal fusion, joint replacement, and carpal tunnel release. Amputation is a radical treatment for severe trauma, infection, gangrene, cancer, ischemia or vascular disease, deformity, or burns. The most common form of amputation is the closed (flap) amputation, in which skin and tissue is used to close the stump. A second, uncommon amputation technique is the open (guillotine) amputation, in which the surgeon cuts through skin, tissue, and bone and a second procedure is required to close and form the stump. See *Common amputation sites and levels*, page 136, for specific body parts affected.

Preoperative preparation

Nursing diagnosis

Fear related to surgical procedure, change in life-style, and resulting disability

COMMON AMPUTATION SITES AND LEVELS

• *Partial foot:* removal of one or more toes and part of the foot
• *Total foot:* removal of the foot below the ankle joint
• *Ankle (Syme's amputation):* removal of the foot at the ankle joint
• *Below-the-knee:* removal of the leg 5″ to 7″ (12.7 to 17.8 cm) below the knee.
• *Knee disarticulation:* removal of the patella with the quadriceps brought over the end of the femur, or fixation of the patella to a cut surface between the condyles (known as the Gritti-Stokes operation)
• *Above-the-knee:* removal of the leg from 3″ (7.6 cm) above the knee

• *Hip disarticulation:* removal of both the leg and hip, or the leg and a portion of the pelvis
• *Hemipelvectomy:* removal of a leg and half of the pelvis
• *Fingers:* removal of one or more fingers at the hinge or condyloid joints
• *Wrist disarticulation:* removal of the hand at the wrist
• *Below-the-elbow:* removal of the lower arm about 7″ (17.8 cm) below the elbow
• *Elbow disarticulation:* removal of the lower arm at the elbow
• *Above-the-elbow:* removal of the arm from 3″ (7.6 cm) above the elbow

Desired outcome: The patient will verbalize an understanding of the anticipated postoperative events and discuss his concerns.

Interventions
Review the doctor's explanation of the procedure with the patient and answer any questions he may have.
Rationale: The patient faces not only a surgical procedure but also the loss of a body part, change in mobility, and possibly a change in the ability to perform his job. Because of his anxieties, the patient may require extensive discussions about postoperative events before he can understand and begin to accept them.

Nursing diagnosis
Knowledge Deficit related to surgical procedure, surgical outcome, and postsurgical rehabilitation
Desired outcome: The patient will verbalize an understanding of the procedure and postsurgical rehabilitation.

Interventions
1. Assess the patient's understanding of the procedure. Be sure to consult with the patient's nurse or your instructor before doing so; you may wish to have one or both present during your initial visit. Become familiar with the surgeon's and institution's routine measures for postoperative care and rehabilitation, such as postoperative exercises to strengthen the remaining limb and procedures for fitting a prosthesis.
Rationale: Anxiety often impairs comprehension; denial may prevent the patient from recognizing the need for this information. You may need to repeat preoperative teaching.
2. Discuss the phenomenon of "phantom" pain, itching, or tingling at the amputation site. Explain that such sensations often occur but are transient.

Rationale: Knowing what to expect may cause the patient some worry but should also decrease postoperative panic and depression. Avoid specific time frames for recovery and prosthesis fitting so the patient will not compare himself with others. Recovery varies among individuals.

Postoperative care (immediate)
See "General postoperative period," page 31, in Section 2.

Nursing diagnosis
Altered Comfort: Pain related to surgical amputation and phantom pain
Desired outcome: The patient will verbalize pain relief.

Interventions
1. Elevate the stump on a pillow or other support for 24 to 48 hours postoperatively, or as ordered.
Rationale: Stump elevation may reduce swelling and thus reduce pain. Be aware of the possibility of contractures, however, and change the position of the affected leg every 2 hours.
2. Provide analgesics and other pain control measures, such as heat application and whirlpool therapy, as ordered. (In some hospitals, this is done by a physical therapist.)
Rationale: Pain increases anxiety and interferes with the patient's ability to walk and perform exercises. Severe, unremitting pain may point to infection.
3. Keep the stump wrapped with elastic bandages. Rewrap the stump twice a day or as ordered. Always check with the surgeon for specific dressing requirements, such as an elastic stump stocking.
Rationale: A properly applied bandage is essential to support soft tissue, control edema and pain, and mold the stump to enable proper fitting of a prosthesis.

Nursing diagnosis
Impaired Physical Mobility related to altered gait
Desired outcome: The patient will walk and perform prescribed exercises.

Interventions
1. Instruct the patient in proper body alignment, and teach him not to prop the stump after the first 48 hours postoperatively.
Rationale: These measures can help prevent stump contractures and deformity.
2. Encourage the patient to walk frequently, if possible, or, if not possible, to perform active or passive range-of-motion exercises. (*Note:* Always check the surgeon's orders and consult a physical therapist before initiating any such measures.)
Rationale: These measures can help prevent contractures and other postoperative complications.

Nursing diagnosis

Grieving related to loss of limb and effects on life-style
Desired outcome: The patient will verbalize his feelings.

Interventions

1. Encourage the patient to express his feelings and to resume an independent life-style as soon as possible after surgery. Enlist the support of the patient's family and friends and possibly the institution's social services department in this effort.
Rationale: Encouragement and support can help motivate the patient toward recovery.
2. Have the patient meet with home health care personnel while in the hospital, if possible.
Rationale: A visit from home health care personnel can help the patient anticipate environmental changes that may be required in the home.

Nursing diagnosis

Potential Disturbance in Self-Concept related to loss of body part
Desired outcome: The patient will express a positive self-image.

Interventions

1. Provide the patient with information about prostheses, as appropriate. (Although this is normally done by the physical therapist, the patient may have additional questions you can answer.)
Rationale: A prosthesis will enhance the patient's total self-concept and aid him in resuming an independent life-style.
2. Instruct the patient in proper stump care. Encourage the patient to participate in his care, if possible, or arrange for home care if necessary.
Rationale: Participation will encourage acceptance of the amputation and of the prosthesis.

6 Medications

Use of certain medications—both currently and in the recent past—may put your patient at risk for complications during the perioperative period. Some drugs can reduce resistance to infection by interfering with the immune system. For example, use of corticosteroids (such as prednisone), immunosuppressive drugs (such as cyclophosphamide), and long-term antibiotics is associated with increased fungal and bacterial infections usually not encountered postoperatively. Other drugs, including insulin, cardiovascular drugs (such as digitalis), and neurologic-psychotropic drugs, may require discontinuation or dosage adjustments throughout the perioperative period.

Because of the potential for serious complications, you'll need to pay particular attention to your patient's drug history—especially his use of any of the medications listed above—during the perioperative period. Be sure to report any such drug use immediately.

☐ Antibiotics

Antibiotics may be used preoperatively to combat anticipated infection during the operative period, especially when the risk of infection is significant or when the consequences of infection are extremely serious, as in surgical procedures involving vascular, cardiac, or joint prostheses.

Prophylactic antibiotics, usually administered 2 hours before surgery (unless the patient has an old infection in the operative site, in which case antibiotics may be administered earlier), may be discontinued a few hours after the procedure. The specific antibiotic chosen depends on the surgical procedure and the patient's condition. For example, in urologic surgery, the antibiotic used is based on the patient's urine culture. In colon surgery, antibiotics are given prophylactically to fight anticipated wound infection from anaerobic bacteria.

Systemic antibiotics are used to treat postoperative wound infections. The specific antibiotic chosen may be based on results of a wound culture from a significant specimen or may be the drug of choice currently used to treat a particular infection.

Below are selected antibiotics commonly prescribed during the perioperative period. (*Note:* Italicized adverse reactions are common or life-threatening.)

Amikacin (Amikin)

General
Availability: Rx.
Pregnancy risk category: C.

Classification
Pharmacologic: aminoglycoside.
Therapeutic: antibacterial.

Pharmacokinetics
Half-life: 2 to 2½ hours in normal renal function; up to 150 hours in renal impairment.
Excretion: by kidneys as unchanged drug.

Indications and dosage
• Serious infections caused by sensitive *Pseudomonas aeruginosa, Escherichia coli, Proteus, Klebsiella, Serratia, Enterobacter, Acinetobacter, Providencia, Citrobacter, Staphylococcus. Adults and children with normal renal function:* 15 mg/kg/day divided q 8 to 12 hours I.M. or I.V. infusion (in 100 to 200 ml dextrose 5% in water over 30 to 60 minutes). May be given by direct I.V. push if necessary.
• Meningitis. *Adults:* systemic therapy as above; may also use up to 20 mg intrathecally or intraventricularly daily.
• Uncomplicated urinary tract infections. *Adults:* 250 mg I.M. or I.V. b.i.d. *Adults with renal impairment:* initially, 7.5 mg/kg. Subsequent doses and frequency determined by serum amikacin levels and renal function studies.

Contraindications and cautions
• Contraindicated in aminoglycoside sensitivity.
• Use cautiously in elderly patients and in those with renal impairment, dehydration, cranial nerve VIII damage, myasthenia gravis, or Parkinson's disease.

Adverse reactions
CNS: headache, lethargy, neuromuscular blockade.
EENT: ototoxicity (tinnitus, vertigo, hearing loss).
GU: nephrotoxicity (cells or casts in urine, oliguria, proteinuria, decreased creatinine clearance, increased blood urea nitrogen [BUN] and serum creatinine levels).

Interactions
Cephalothin: increased nephrotoxicity. Use together cautiously.
Dimenhydrinate: possible masked symptoms of ototoxicity. Use cautiously.
I.V. loop diuretics (such as furosemide): increased ototoxicity. Use cautiously.
Other aminoglycosides, amphotericin B, cisplatin, methoxyflurane: possible increased nephrotoxicity. Use together cautiously.
Parenteral penicillins (carbenicillin, ticarcillin): amikacin inactivation. Don't mix together in I.V. line.

Patient-teaching tips
Tell patient to notify doctor if he develops tinnitus, vertigo, or hearing loss.

Special considerations
• Obtain specimens for culture and sensitivity testing before first dose. Therapy may begin pending results.
• Weigh patient and obtain baseline renal function studies before therapy.
• Evaluate patient's hearing before and during therapy.
• Monitor renal function (output, specific gravity, urinalysis, BUN and creatinine levels, and creatinine clearance). Notify doctor of signs of deteriorating renal function.
• Ensure adequate hydration during therapy.
• Watch for signs of superinfection.
• Don't collect blood in a heparinized tube.
• Draw blood for peak amikacin level 1 hour after I.M. injection and 30 to 60 minutes after infusion; for trough levels, draw blood just before next dose. Peak serum levels above 35 mcg/ml and trough levels above 10 mcg/ml may be associated with higher incidence of toxicity.
• Usual duration of therapy is 7 to 10 days. If no response after 3 to 5 days, therapy may be stopped and new specimens obtained for culture and sensitivity studies.
• Potency isn't affected if solution turns light yellow.
• After infusion, flush line with normal saline solution or dextrose 5% in water.

Amoxicillin (Amoxil, Trimox)

General
Availability: Rx.
Pregnancy risk category: B.

Classification
Pharmacologic: aminopenicillin.
Therapeutic: antibacterial.

Pharmacokinetics
Half-life: 60 to 80 minutes.
Oral absorption: 75% to 90%.
Excretion: by kidneys, mainly unchanged.

Indications and dosage
• Systemic infections, acute and chronic urinary tract infections caused by susceptible strains of gram-positive and gram-negative organisms. *Adults:* 750 mg to 1.5 g P.O. daily, divided into doses given q 8 hours.
• Uncomplicated gonorrhea. *Adults:* 3 g P.O. with 1 g probenecid given as a single dose.
• Uncomplicated urinary tract infections caused by susceptible organisms. *Adults:* 3 g P.O. given as a single dose.

Contraindications and cautions

• Use cautiously in patients with other drug allergies, especially to cephalosporins (possible cross-allergenicity).
• Also use cautiously in patients with mononucleosis because of a high incidence of maculopapular rash.

Adverse reactions

Blood: anemia, thrombocytopenia, thrombocytopenic purpura, eosinophilia, leukopenia.
GI: nausea, vomiting, *diarrhea.*
Other: hypersensitivity (erythematous maculopapular rash, urticaria, anaphylaxis), overgrowth of nonsusceptible organisms.

Interactions

Probenecid: increased amoxicillin levels. Probenecid is often used for this purpose.

Patient-teaching tips

• Tell patient to take medication exactly as prescribed, even after he feels better. Entire quantity prescribed should be taken.
• Warn patient never to use leftover penicillin for a new illness or to share penicillin with family and friends.
• Instruct patient to call the doctor if rash, fever, or chills develop. Rash, the most common allergic reaction, affects patients taking allopurinol most frequently.

Special considerations

• Before giving amoxicillin, ask patient if he's had any allergic reactions to penicillin. However, a negative history of penicillin allergy doesn't rule out a future allergic reaction.
• Obtain specimens for culture and sensitivity tests before first dose. Unnecessary to wait for results before beginning therapy.
• Give amoxicillin at least 1 hour before bacteriostatic antibiotics.
• Give drug with food to prevent GI distress.
• Large doses may cause increased yeast growths.
• Urine glucose determination may be false-positive with copper sulfate tests (Clinitest); glucose-enzymatic tests (Clinistix, Tes-Tape) aren't affected.
• With prolonged therapy, bacterial and fungal superinfection may occur, especially in elderly or debilitated patients or those with low resistance to infection. Close observation essential.
• Trimox oral suspension may be stored at room temperature for up to 2 weeks. Be sure to check product labels for storage information.
• Amoxicillin and ampicillin have similar clinical applications.
• Amoxicillin appears in breast milk.

Ampicillin (Amcill, Principen)

General

Availability: Rx.
Pregnancy risk category: B.

Classification
Pharmacologic: aminopenicillin.
Therapeutic: antibacterial.

Pharmacokinetics
Half-life: 1 to 1½ hours.
Oral absorption: 35% to 50%.
Excretion: by kidneys, mainly unchanged.

Indications and dosage
• Systemic infections, acute and chronic urinary tract infections caused by susceptible strains of gram-positive and gram-negative organisms. *Adults:* 1 to 4 g P.O. daily, divided into doses given q 6 hours; 2 to 12 g I.M. or I.V. daily, divided into doses given q 4 to 6 hours.
• Meningitis. *Adults:* 8 to 14 g I.V. daily for 3 days, then I.M. divided q 3 to 4 hours.
• Uncomplicated gonorrhea. *Adults:* 3.5 g P.O. with 1 g probenecid given as a single dose.

Contraindications and cautions
• Use cautiously in patients with other drug allergies, especially to cephalosporins (possible cross-allergenicity).
• Also use cautiously in patients with mononucleosis because of the high incidence of maculopapular rash.

Adverse reactions
Blood: anemia, thrombocytopenia, thrombocytopenic purpura, eosinophilia, leukopenia.
GI: nausea, vomiting, *diarrhea,* glossitis, stomatitis.
Local: pain at injection site, vein irritation, thrombophlebitis.
Other: hypersensitivity (erythematous maculopapular rash, urticaria, anaphylaxis), overgrowth of nonsusceptible organisms.

Interactions
Probenecid: increased ampicillin levels. Probenecid is often used for this purpose.

Patient-teaching tips
• Tell patient to take medication exactly as prescribed, even after he feels better. Entire quantity prescribed should be taken.
• Instruct patient to call the doctor if rash, fever, or chills develop. Rash, the most common allergic reaction, occurs most frequently in patients taking allopurinol.
• Warn patient never to use leftover penicillin for a new illness or to share penicillin with family and friends.

Special considerations
• Before giving ampicillin, ask patient if he's had any allergic reactions to penicillin. However, a negative history of penicillin allergy doesn't rule out a future allergic reaction.

• Obtain specimens for culture and sensitivity tests before first dose. Unnecessary to wait for results before beginning therapy.

• When given orally, drug may cause GI disturbances. Food may interfere with absorption, so give 1 to 2 hours before meals or 2 to 3 hours after.

• Don't give I.M. or I.V. unless infection is severe or patient can't take oral dose.

• When giving I.V., mix with dextrose 5% in water or saline solution. Don't mix with other drugs or solutions; they might be incompatible.

• Initial dilution in vial is stable for 1 hour. Follow manufacturer's direction for stability data when ampicillin is further diluted for I.V. infusion.

• Give I.V. intermittently to prevent vein irritation.

• Alter dosage in hepatic and renal impairment.

• Large doses may cause increased yeast growths.

• With prolonged therapy, bacterial or fungal superinfection may occur, especially in elderly or debilitated patients, or in those with low resistance to infection because of immunosuppressive therapy. Close observation is essential.

• Give penicillins at least 1 hour before bacteriostatic antibiotics.

Cefazolin (Ancef, Kefzol)

General
Availability: Rx.
Pregnancy risk category: B.

Classification
Pharmacologic: first-generation cephalosporin.
Therapeutic: antibacterial.

Pharmacokinetics
Half-life: 1½ hours (normal renal function); 3 to 42 hours (impaired renal function).
Excretion: by kidneys, mostly unchanged.

Indications and dosage
Serious infections of respiratory and genitourinary (GU) tracts, skin and soft-tissue infections, bone and joint infections, septicemia, and endocarditis caused by *Escherichia coli, Enterobacteriaceae,* gonococci, group A beta-hemolytic streptococci, *Hemophilus influenzae, Klebsiella, Proteus mirabilis, Staphylococcus aureus,* and *S. pneumoniae;* and for perioperative prophylaxis. *Adults:* 250 mg I.M. or I.V. q 8 hours to 1 g q 6 hours. Maximum 12 g daily in life-threatening situations.

Total daily dosage is same for I.M. or I.V. administration and depends on susceptibility of organism and severity of infection. In patients with impaired renal function, doses or frequency of administration must be modified according to degree of renal impairment, severity of infection, and susceptibility of organism.

Contraindications and cautions
• Contraindicated in hypersensitivity to other cephalosporins.
• Use cautiously in patients with renal impairment and in those with history of sensitivity to penicillin.

Adverse reactions
Blood: transient neutropenia, leukopenia, eosinophilia, anemia.
CNS: dizziness, headache, malaise, paresthesias.
GI: pseudomembranous colitis, nausea, anorexia, vomiting, *diarrhea,* glossitis, dyspepsia, abdominal cramps, anal pruritus, tenesmus, oral candidiasis (thrush).
GU: genital pruritus and moniliasis, vaginitis.
Skin: maculopapular and erythematous rashes, urticaria.
Local: at injection site—pain, induration, sterile abscesses, tissue sloughing; phlebitis and thrombophlebitis with I.V. injection.
Other: hypersensitivity, dyspnea.

Interactions
Probenecid: possible inhibited excretion and increased blood levels of cefazolin. Probenecid may be used for this purpose.

Patient-teaching tips
Tell patient to report any unusual reactions to the doctor.

Special considerations
• Before giving drug, ask patient if he's had a previous allergic reaction to penicillins or cephalosporins. However, a negative history doesn't rule out a future allergic reaction.
• Obtain specimens for culture and sensitivity tests before first dose. Don't wait for results before initiating therapy.
• Not as painful as other cephalosporins when given I.M.
• Inject deep I.M. into a large muscle mass, such as gluteus or lateral aspect of thigh.
• Alternate injection sites if I.V. therapy lasts longer than 3 days. Use of small I.V. needles in the larger available veins may be preferable.
• Prolonged use may cause overgrowth of nonsusceptible organisms. Monitor patient for signs of superinfection.
• Avoid dosages greater than 4 g daily in patients with severe renal impairment.
• About 40% to 75% of patients receiving cephalosporins show a false-positive direct Coombs' test; only a few of these indicate hemolytic anemia.
• Urine glucose determinations may be false-positive with copper sulfate tests (Clinitest); glucose oxidase tests (Clinistix, Tes-Tape) aren't affected.
• Cefazolin appears in breast milk.

Cefoperazone (Cefobid)

General
Availability: Rx.
Pregnancy risk category: B.

Classification
Pharmacologic: third-generation cephalosporin.
Therapeutic: antibacterial.

Pharmacokinetics
Half-life: 1½ to 2½ hours (normal renal function); 3 to 4 hours (impaired renal function).
Excretion: in feces, mainly unchanged.

Indications and dosage
Serious infections of the respiratory tract; intraabdominal, gynecologic, and skin infections; bacteremia; septicemia. Susceptible microorganisms include *Bacteroides fragilis, Citrobacter, Enterobacter,* enterococci, *Escherichia coli, Hemophilus influenzae, Klebsiella, Proteus,* some *Pseudomonas* species including *Pseudomonas aeruginosa, Staphylococcus aureus* (penicillinase- and nonpenicillinase-producing), *Staphylococcus epidermidis, Streptococcus pneumoniae,* and *Streptococcus pyogenes. Adults:* usual dose is 1 to 2 g q 12 hours I.M. or I.V.

In severe infections, or infections caused by less sensitive organisms, the total daily dosage or frequency may be increased up to 16 g daily. Usually no dosage adjustment is necessary in patients with renal impairment. However, dosages of 4 g daily should be given very cautiously in patients with hepatic disease.

Contraindications and cautions
• Contraindicated in hypersensitivity to other cephalosporins.
• Use cautiously in patients with impaired renal function and in those with history of sensitivity to penicillin.

Adverse reactions
Blood: transient neutropenia, eosinophilia, hemolytic anemia, *hypoprothrombinemia, bleeding.*
CNS: headache, malaise, paresthesias, dizziness.
GI: pseudomembranous colitis, nausea, anorexia, vomiting, *diarrhea,* glossitis, dyspepsia, abdominal cramps, tenesmus, anal pruritus, oral candidiasis (thrush).
GU: genital pruritus and moniliasis.
Hepatic: mildly elevated liver enzymes.
Skin: maculopapular and erythematous rashes, urticaria.
Local: at injection site—pain, induration, sterile abscesses, temperature elevation, tissue sloughing; phlebitis and thrombophlebitis with I.V. injection.
Other: hypersensitivity, dyspnea.

Interactions
Probenecid: possible inhibited excretion and increased blood levels of cefoperazone. Probenecid may be used for this purpose.
Ethyl alcohol: possible disulfiram-like reaction. Warn patients not to drink alcohol for several days after discontinuing cefoperazone.

Patient-teaching tips
Tell patient to report any unusual reactions to the doctor.

Special considerations
• Before giving drug, ask patient if he's had a previous allergic reaction to penicillins or cephalosporins. However, a negative history doesn't rule out a future allergic reaction.
• Obtain specimens for culture and sensitivity tests before first dose. Don't wait for results before initiating therapy.
• Inject deep I.M. into a large muscle mass, such as gluteus or lateral aspect of the thigh.
• Because of high degree of biliary excretion, drug may cause diarrhea more commonly than other cephalosporins.
• Prolonged use may cause overgrowth of nonsusceptible organisms. Monitor patient for signs of superinfection.
• Drug's chemical structure includes the methyltetrazole side chain, which has been associated with bleeding disorders. If bleeding occurs, give vitamin K.
• Cefoperazone possesses greater activity than first-generation cephalosporins against gram-negative organisms, but less activity against gram-positive organisms.
• Urine glucose determinations may be false-positive with copper sulfate tests (Clinitest); glucose oxidase tests (Clinistix, Tes-Tape) aren't affected.
• Cefoperazone appears in breast milk.

Cefoxitin (Mefoxin)

General
Availability: Rx.
Pregnancy risk category: B.

Classification
Pharmacologic: second-generation cephalosporin.
Therapeutic: antibacterial.

Pharmacokinetics
Half-life: 42 to 66 minutes (normal renal function); 2 to 20 hours (impaired renal function).
Excretion: by kidneys, mainly unchanged.

Indications and dosage
Serious infection of respiratory and GU tracts, skin and soft-tissue infections, bone and joint infections, intraabdominal infections, and septicemia caused by *Bacteroides* species, including *B.*

fragilis, Escherichia coli and other coliform bacteria, *Hemophilus influenzae, Klebsiella, Staphylococcus aureus* (penicillinase- and nonpenicillinase-producing), *Staphylococcus epidermidis,* and streptococci. *Adults:* 1 to 2 g q 6 to 8 hours for uncomplicated infection. Up to 12 g daily in life-threatening infections.

Total daily dosage is same for I.M. or I.V. administration and depends on susceptibility of organism and severity of infection. In patients with renal impairment, doses or frequency of administration must be modified according to degree of renal impairment, severity of infection, and susceptibility of organism.

Contraindications and cautions
• Contraindicated in hypersensitivity to other cephalosporins.
• Use cautiously in patients with renal impairment and in those with history of sensitivity to penicillin.

Adverse reactions
Blood: transient neutropenia, eosinophilia, hemolytic anemia.
CNS: headache, malaise, paresthesias, dizziness.
GI: pseudomembranous colitis, nausea, anorexia, vomiting, *diarrhea,* glossitis, dyspepsia, abdominal cramps, tenesmus, anal pruritus, oral candidiasis (thrush).
GU: genital pruritus and moniliasis.
Skin: maculopapular and erythematous rashes, urticaria.
Local: at injection site—pain, induration, sterile abscesses, tissue sloughing; phlebitis and thrombophlebitis with I.V. injection.
Other: hypersensitivity, dyspnea, fever.

Interactions
Probenecid: possible inhibited excretion and increased cefoxitin blood levels. Probenecid may be used for this purpose.

Patient-teaching tips
Tell patient to report any unusual reactions to the doctor.

Special considerations
• Before giving drug, ask patient if he's had a previous allergic reaction to penicillins or cephalosporins. However, a negative history doesn't rule out a future allergic reaction.
• Obtain specimens for culture and sensitivity tests before first dose. Don't wait for results before initiating therapy.
• Inject deep I.M. into a large muscle mass, such as gluteus or lateral aspect of thigh.
• Associated with development of thrombophlebitis. Assess I.V. site frequently.
• Prolonged use may cause overgrowth of nonsusceptible organisms. Monitor patient for superinfection.
• Useful when anaerobic or mixed aerobic-anaerobic infection is suspected, especially *Bacteroides fragilis.*
• Urine glucose determinations may be false-positive with copper sulfate tests (Clinitest); glucose oxidase tests (Clinistix, Tes-Tape) aren't affected.

• For I.V. use, reconstitute 1 g with at least 10 ml of sterile water for injection, and 2 g with 10 to 20 ml. Solutions of dextrose 5% and 0.9% sodium chloride for injection can also be used.
• Reconstitute I.M. injection with 0.5% or 1% lidocaine hydrochloride (without epinephrine) to minimize pain.
• After reconstitution, drug remains stable for 24 hours at room temperature or 1 week under refrigeration.
• Cefoxitin appears in breast milk.

Ceftazidime (Fortaz)

General
Availability: Rx.
Pregnancy risk category: B.

Classification
Pharmacologic: third-generation cephalosporin.
Therapeutic: antibacterial.

Pharmacokinetics
Half-life: almost 2 hours.
Excretion: by kidneys, almost entirely unchanged.

Indications and dosage
Serious infections of the urinary and lower respiratory tracts; gynecologic, intraabdominal, CNS, and skin infections; bacteremia; and septicemia. Susceptible microorganisms include some strains of *Bacteroides* species, *Enterobacter, Escherichia coli, Hemophilus influenzae, Klebsiella, Proteus, Pseudomonas, Staphylococcus aureus* (penicillinase- and nonpenicillinase-producing), and streptococci, including *Streptococcus pneumoniae* and *Streptococcus pyogenes. Adults:* 1 g I.V. or I.M. q 8 to 12 hours; up to 6 g daily in life-threatening infections.
    Total daily dosage is same for I.M. or I.V. administration and depends on susceptibility of organism and severity of infection. In patients with renal impairment, doses or frequency of administration must be modified according to degree of renal impairment, severity of infection, and susceptibility of organism.

Contraindications and cautions
• Contraindicated in cephalosporin hypersensitivity.
• Use cautiously in patients with history of sensitivity to penicillin.

Adverse reactions
Blood: eosinophilia, thrombocytosis, leukopenia.
CNS: headache, dizziness.
GI: pseudomembranous enterocolitis, nausea, vomiting, diarrhea, dysgeusia, abdominal cramps.
GU: genital pruritus and moniliasis.
Hepatic: transient elevation of liver enzymes.
Skin: maculopapular and erythematous rashes, urticaria.

Local: at injection site—pain, induration, sterile abscesses, tissue sloughing; phlebitis and thrombophlebitis with I.V. injection.
Other: hypersensitivity, dyspnea, elevated temperature.

Interactions
Sodium bicarbonate-containing solutions: instability of ceftazidime. Don't mix together.

Patient-teaching tips
Tell patient to report any unusual reactions to the doctor.

Special considerations
• Before giving drug, ask patient if he's had a previous allergic reaction to penicillins or cephalosporins. However, a negative history doesn't rule out a future allergic reaction.
• Obtain specimens for culture and sensitivity tests before first dose. Don't wait for results before initiating therapy.
• Inject deep I.M. into a large muscle mass, such as gluteus or lateral aspect of thigh.
• Prolonged use may cause overgrowth of nonsusceptible organisms. Monitor patient for signs of superinfection.
• Vials of ceftazidime are supplied under reduced pressure. When the antibiotic is dissolved, CO_2 is released and positive pressure develops. Each brand of ceftazidime includes specific instructions for reconstitution. Read and follow these instructions carefully.
• This third-generation cephalosporin has excellent activity against infections caused by *Pseudomonas aeruginosa.* May be prescribed for these infections, especially when aminoglycosides are potentially too dangerous.
• Ceftazidime appears in breast milk.

Ceftizoxime (Cefizox)

General
Availability: Rx.
Pregnancy risk category: B.

Classification
Pharmacologic: third-generation cephalosporin.
Therapeutic: antibacterial.

Pharmacokinetics
Half-life: 1⅔ hours (normal renal function); 30 hours (impaired renal function).
Excretion: by kidneys, mostly unchanged.

Indications and dosage
Serious infections of the urinary and lower respiratory tracts; gynecologic, intraabdominal, bone and joint, and skin infections; bacteremia; septicemia; and meningitis. Susceptible microorganisms include *Enterobacter, Escherichia coli, Hemophilus influen-*

zae, Klebsiella, Peptostreptococcus, Proteus, some *Pseudomonas*
species, *Staphylococcus aureus* (penicillinase- and nonpenicillinase-producing), *Staphylococcus epidermidis,* and streptococci,
including *Streptococcus pneumoniae* and *Streptococcus pyogenes. Adults:* 1 to 2 g I.V. or I.M. q 8 to 12 hours. In life-
threatening infections, up to 2 g q 4 hours.
 Total daily dosage is same for I.M. or I.V. administration and
depends on susceptibility of organism and severity of infection.
In patients with renal impairment, doses or frequency of administration must be modified according to degree of renal impairment, severity of infection, and susceptibility of organism.

Contraindications and cautions
• Contraindicated in cephalosporin hypersensitivity.
• Use cautiously in patients with renal impairment and in those
with history of sensitivity to penicillin.

Adverse reactions
Blood: transient neutropenia, eosinophilia, hemolytic anemia.
CNS: headache, malaise, paresthesias, dizziness.
GI: pseudomembranous colitis, nausea, anorexia, vomiting, *diar-
rhea,* glossitis, dyspepsia, abdominal cramps, tenesmus, anal pru-
ritus.
GU: genital pruritus and moniliasis.
Skin: maculopapular and erythematous rashes, urticaria.
*Local: at injection site—pain, induration, sterile abscesses, tissue
sloughing; phlebitis and thrombophlebitis with I.V. injection.*
Other: hypersensitivity, dyspnea, fever.

Interactions
Probenecid: possible inhibited excretion and increased blood
levels of ceftizoxime. Probenecid may be used for this purpose.

Patient-teaching tips
Tell patient to report any unusual reactions to the doctor.

Special considerations
• Before giving drug, ask patient if he's had a previous allergic
reaction to penicillins or cephalosporins. However, a negative
history doesn't rule out a future allergic reaction.
• Obtain specimens for culture and sensitivity tests before first
dose. Don't wait for results before initiating therapy.
• Inject deep I.M. into a large muscle mass, such as gluteus or
lateral aspect of thigh.
• Prolonged use may cause overgrowth of nonsusceptible organisms. Monitor patient for signs of superinfection.
• Ceftizoxime is comparable in activity to cefotaxime, moxalactam,
ceftriaxone, and cefoperazone. No significant degree of bleeding or
disulfiram-type reaction has been reported with its use.
• Drug appears in breast milk.

Ceftriaxone (Rocephin)

General
Availability: Rx.
Pregnancy risk category: B.

Classification
Pharmacologic: third-generation cephalosporin.
Therapeutic: antibacterial.

Pharmacokinetics
Half-life: 4½ to 9 hours (normal renal function); 12 to 16 hours (impaired renal function).
Metabolism: partially metabolized in liver.
Excretion: by kidneys as unchanged and inactive metabolites.

Indications and dosage
• Serious infections of the urinary and lower respiratory tracts; gynecologic, intraabdominal, and skin infections; bacteremia; and septicemia. Susceptible microorganisms include *Enterobacter, Escherichia coli, Hemophilus influenzae, Klebsiella, Peptostreptococcus, Proteus, Pseudomonas, Staphylococcus aureus* (penicillinase- and nonpenicillinase-producing), *Staphylococcus epidermidis, Streptococcus pneumoniae,* and *Streptococcus pyogenes. Adults:* 1 to 2 g I.M. or I.V. once daily or b.i.d. in equally divided doses. Total daily dosage shouldn't exceed 4 g.
• Meningitis. *Adults:* 100 mg/kg in divided doses q 12 hours. May give loading dose of 75 mg/kg.
   Total daily dosage is same for I.M. or I.V. administration and depends on susceptibility of organism and severity of infection.

Contraindications and cautions
• Contraindicated in hypersensitivity to other cephalosporins.
• Use cautiously in patients with history of sensitivity to penicillin.

Adverse reactions
Blood: eosinophilia, thrombocytosis, leukopenia.
CNS: headache, dizziness.
GI: pseudomembranous enterocolitis, nausea, vomiting, diarrhea, dysgeusia, abdominal cramps.
GU: genital pruritus and moniliasis.
Hepatic: transient elevation in liver enzymes.
Skin: maculopapular and erythematous rashes, urticaria.
Local: at injection site—pain, induration, sterile abscesses, tissue sloughing; phlebitis and thrombophlebitis with I.V. injection.
Other: hypersensitivity, dyspnea, fever.

Interactions
Probenecid: possible inhibited excretion and increased ceftriaxone blood levels. Probenecid may be used for this purpose.

Patient-teaching tips
Tell patient to report any unusual reactions to the doctor.

Special considerations
• Before giving drug, ask patient if he's had a previous allergic reaction to penicillins or cephalosporins. However, a negative history doesn't rule out a future allergic reaction.
• Obtain specimens for culture and sensitivity tests before first dose. Don't wait for results before initiating therapy.
• Inject deep I.M. into a large muscle mass, such as gluteus or lateral aspect of thigh.
• Prolonged use may cause overgrowth of nonsusceptible organisms. Monitor patient for signs of superinfection.
• Dosage adjustment generally not needed in patients with renal insufficiency.
• Becoming quite popular in home antibiotic programs for outpatient treatment of serious infections, such as osteomyelitis.
• Ceftriaxone appears in breast milk.

Cefuroxime (Kefurox)
General
Availability: Rx.
Pregnancy risk category: B.

Classification
Pharmacologic: second-generation cephalosporin.
Therapeutic: antibacterial.

Pharmacokinetics
Half-life: 1⅓ hours (normal renal function); 15 to 22 hours (impaired renal function).
Excretion: by kidneys, mostly unchanged.

Indications and dosage
Serious infections of the urinary and lower respiratory tracts, skin and skin structure infections, septicemia, meningitis, and gonorrhea. Susceptible organisms include *Enterobacter, Escherichia coli, Hemophilus influenzae, Klebsiella, Neisseria gonorrhoeae, Staphylococcus aureus, Streptococcus pneumoniae,* and *Streptococcus pyogenes. Adults:* 750 mg to 1.5 g I.M. or I.V. q 8 hours, usually for 5 to 10 days. For life-threatening infections and infections caused by less susceptible organisms, 1.5 g I.M. or I.V. q 6 hours; for bacterial meningitis, up to 3 g I.V. q 6 hours.

Total daily dosage is same for I.M. or I.V. administration and depends on susceptibility of organism and severity of infection. In patients with renal impairment, doses or frequency of administration must be modified according to degree of renal impairment, severity of infection, susceptibility of organism, and blood levels of drug.

Contraindications and cautions
• Contraindicated in hypersensitivity to other cephalosporins.
• Use cautiously in patients with renal impairment and in those with history of sensitivity to penicillin.

Adverse reactions
Blood: transient neutropenia, eosinophilia, hemolytic anemia, decrease in hemoglobin and hematocrit levels.
CNS: headache, malaise, paresthesias, dizziness.
GI: pseudomembranous colitis, nausea, anorexia, vomiting, *diarrhea,* glossitis, dyspepsia, abdominal cramps, tenesmus, anal pruritus.
GU: genital pruritus and moniliasis.
Skin: maculopapular and erythematous rashes, urticaria.
Local: at injection site—pain, induration, sterile abscesses, warmth, tissue sloughing; phlebitis and thrombophlebitis with I.V. injection.
Other: hypersensitivity, dyspnea.

Interactions
Probenecid: possible inhibited excretion and increased blood levels of cefuroxime. Probenecid may be used for this purpose.

Patient-teaching tips
Tell patient to report any unusual reactions to the doctor.

Special considerations
• Before giving drug, ask patient if he's had a previous allergic reaction to penicillins or cephalosporins. However, a negative history doesn't rule out a future allergic reaction.
• Obtain specimens for culture and sensitivity tests before first dose. Don't wait for results before initiating therapy.
• Inject deep I.M. into a large muscle mass, such as gluteus or lateral aspect of thigh.
• Prolonged use may cause overgrowth of nonsusceptible organisms. Monitor patient for signs of superinfection.
• Unlike some other cephalosporins, cefuroxime hasn't been associated with prothrombin deficiency and bleeding. Advantage over cefamandole: Cefuroxime is useful in treating meningitis.
• Cefuroxime appears in breast milk.

Cephalexin (Keflex)

General
Availability: Rx.
Pregnancy risk category: B.

Classification
Pharmacologic: first-generation cephalosporin.
Therapeutic: antibacterial.

Pharmacokinetics
Half-life: 1 hour (normal renal function); 5 to 30 hours (impaired renal function).
Excretion: by kidneys, mostly unchanged.

Indications and dosage
Infections of respiratory or GU tract, skin and soft tissues, and bone and joints, and otitis media caused by *Escherichia coli* and other coliform bacteria, group A beta-hemolytic streptococci, *Hemophilus influenzae, Klebsiella, Proteus mirabilis, Streptococcus pneumoniae,* and staphylococci. *Adults:* 250 mg to 1 g P.O. q 6 hours.

Contraindications and cautions
• Contraindicated in cephalosporin hypersensitivity.
• Use cautiously in patients with renal impairment and in those with history of sensitivity to penicillin.

Adverse reactions
Blood: transient neutropenia, eosinophilia, anemia.
CNS: dizziness, headache, malaise, paresthesias.
GI: pseudomembranous colitis, nausea, anorexia, vomiting, *diarrhea,* glossitis, dyspepsia, abdominal cramps, anal pruritus, tenesmus, oral candidiasis (thrush).
GU: genital pruritus and moniliasis, vaginitis.
Skin: maculopapular and erythematous rashes, urticaria.
Other: hypersensitivity, dyspnea.

Interactions
Probenecid: possible increased cephalexin blood levels. Probenecid may be used for this purpose.

Patient-teaching tips
• Instruct patient to take medication exactly as prescribed, even after he feels better. Group A beta-hemolytic streptococcal infections should be treated for at least 10 days.
• Tell him to take with food or milk to lessen GI discomfort.
• Warn patient to call doctor if rash develops.

Special considerations
• Before giving drug, ask patient if he's had a previous allergic reaction to penicillins or cephalosporins. However, a negative history doesn't rule out a future allergic reaction.
• Obtain specimens for culture and sensitivity tests before first dose. Don't wait for results before initiating therapy.
• Prolonged use may cause overgrowth of nonsusceptible organisms. Monitor the patient for signs of superinfection.
• Urine glucose determinations may be false-positive with copper sulfate tests (Clinitest); glucose oxidase tests (Clinistix, Tes-Tape) aren't affected.
• To prepare oral suspension: Add required amount of water to powder in two portions. Shake well after each addition. After

mixing, store in refrigerator. Stable for 14 days without significant loss of potency. Keep tightly closed and shake well before using.

Clindamycin (Cleocin)

General
Availability: Rx.
Pregnancy risk category: D.

Classification
Pharmacologic: lincomycin derivative.
Therapeutic: antibacterial.

Pharmacokinetics
Half-life: 2 to 3 hours.
Metabolism: to active and inactive metabolites in liver.
Excretion: in urine and feces.

Indications and dosage
Infections caused by *Bacteroides, Clostridium perfringens, Fusobacterium,* pneumococci, staphylococci, streptococci, and other sensitive aerobic and anaerobic organisms. *Adults:* 150 to 450 mg P.O. q 6 hours; or 300 mg I.M. or I.V. q 6, 8, or 12 hours. Up to 2,700 mg I.M. or I.V. daily, divided q 6, 8, or 12 hours. May be used for severe infections.

Contraindications and cautions
• Contraindicated in patients with known hypersensitivity to the antibiotic congener lincomycin, and in patients with a history of GI disease, especially colitis.
• Use cautiously in patients with renal or hepatic disease, asthma, or significant allergies.

Adverse reactions
Blood: transient leukopenia, eosinophilia, thrombocytopenia.
GI: nausea, vomiting, abdominal pain, *diarrhea, pseudomembranous enterocolitis,* esophagitis, flatulence, anorexia, *bloody or tarry stools, dysphagia.*
Hepatic: elevated AST (SGOT), alkaline phosphatase, bilirubin.
Skin: maculopapular rash, urticaria.
Local: pain, induration, *sterile abscess with I.M. injection;* thrombophlebitis, erythema, and pain after I.V. administration.
Other: unpleasant or bitter taste, *anaphylaxis.*

Interactions
Neuromuscular blocking agents: enhanced effects. Use together cautiously.

Patient-teaching tips
• Instruct patient to report adverse effects to the doctor, especially diarrhea. Warn against treating diarrhea himself.

• Advise patient using the capsule form to take drug with a full glass of water to prevent dysphagia.

Special considerations
• Culture and sensitivity test should be performed before treatment and p.r.n.
• Monitor renal, hepatic, and hematopoietic functions during prolonged therapy.
• Give deep I.M. Rotate sites. Warn that I.M. injection may be painful. Doses greater than 600 mg per injection are not recommended.
• I.M. injection may cause creatine phosphokinase levels to rise because of muscle irritation.
• When giving I.V., check site daily for phlebitis and irritation. For I.V. infusion, dilute each 300 mg in 50 ml solution, and give no faster than 30 mg/minute.
• Don't use in meningitis. Drug does not reach cerebrospinal fluid (CSF).
• Don't refrigerate reconstituted oral solution, because it will thicken. Drug is stable for 2 weeks at room temperature.
• Don't give diphenoxylate compound (Lomotil) to treat drug-induced diarrhea. May prolong and worsen diarrhea.
• Clindamycin appears in breast milk.

Co-trimoxazole (sulfamethoxazole-trimethoprim)(Bactrim, Septra)

General
Availability: Rx.
Pregnancy risk category: C (D if near term).

Classification
Pharmacologic: sulfonamide combination drug.
Therapeutic: antibacterial.

Pharmacokinetics
Half-life: 6 to 12 hours (sulfamethoxazole); 8 to 10 hours (trimethoprim).
Metabolism: both components metabolized in liver.
Excretion: by kidneys.

Indications and dosage
• Urinary tract infections and shigellosis. *Adults:* 160 mg trimethoprim and 800 mg sulfamethoxazole q 12 hours for 10 to 14 days in urinary tract infections and for 5 days in shigellosis. For simple cystitis or acute urethral syndrome, one to three double-strength tablets as a single dose.
• *Pneumocystis carinii* pneumonitis. *Adults:* 20 mg/kg trimethoprim and 100 mg/kg sulfamethoxazole daily in equally divided doses q 6 hours for 14 days.

• Chronic bronchitis. *Adults:* 160 mg trimethoprim and 800 mg sulfamethoxazole q 12 hours for 10 to 14 days.

Contraindications and cautions
• Contraindicated in patients with porphyria.
• Use cautiously and in reduced dosages in patients with hepatic or renal impairment and in those with severe allergy or bronchial asthma, G6PD deficiency, or blood dyscrasias.

Adverse reactions
Blood: agranulocytosis, aplastic anemia, megaloblastic anemia, thrombocytopenia, leukopenia, hemolytic anemia.
CNS: headache, mental depression, convulsions, hallucinations.
GI: nausea, vomiting, diarrhea, abdominal pain, anorexia, stomatitis.
GU: toxic nephrosis with oliguria and anuria, crystalluria, hematuria.
Hepatic: jaundice.
Skin: erythema multiforme (Stevens-Johnson syndrome), generalized skin eruption, epidermal necrolysis, exfoliative dermatitis, photosensitivity, urticaria, pruritus.
Other: hypersensitivity, serum sickness, drug fever, anaphylaxis.

Interactions
Ammonium chloride, ascorbic acid: with doses sufficient to acidify urine, possible precipitation of sulfonamide and crystalluria. Don't use together.

Patient-teaching tips
Tell patient to promptly report skin rash, sore throat, fever, or mouth sores—early signs of blood dyscrasias.

Special considerations
• Adverse reactions, especially hypersensitivity, occur much more frequently in patients with acquired immunodeficiency syndrome (AIDS).
• For I.V. infusion, dilute with dextrose 5% in water before administration. Don't mix with other drugs or solutions. Must be used within 2 hours of mixing. Don't refrigerate.
• Give I.V. infusion over 60 to 90 minutes. Don't give by rapid infusion or bolus injection.
• Often used in extremely ill immunosuppressed patients for treatment of *Pneumocystis carinii* pneumonia.
• Oral suspension available.
• Note that the "DS" product means "double strength."
• Used effectively for chronic bacterial prostatitis.
• Used prophylactically for recurrent urinary tract infections in women and for traveler's diarrhea.
• Sulfonamides appear in breast milk.

Dicloxacillin (Dycill)

General
Availability: Rx.
Pregnancy risk category: B.

Classification
Pharmacologic: penicillinase-resistant penicillin.
Therapeutic: antibiotic.

Pharmacokinetics
Half-life: 30 to 60 minutes.
Oral absorption: 37% to 50%.
Excretion: by kidneys as metabolites and unchanged drug.

Indications and dosage
Systemic infections caused by penicillinase-producing staphylococci. *Adults:* 1 to 2 g P.O. daily, divided into doses given q 6 hours.

Contraindications and cautions
• Contraindicated in patients allergic to any other penicillin or to cephalosporins (possible cross-allergenicity).
• Use cautiously in renal impairment; decreased dosage required in moderate to severe renal failure.

Adverse reactions
Blood: eosinophilia.
GI: nausea, vomiting, *epigastric distress,* flatulence, *diarrhea.*
Other: hypersensitivity (pruritus, urticaria, rash, anaphylaxis), overgrowth of nonsusceptible organisms.

Interactions
Probenecid: increased dicloxacillin levels. Probenecid may be used for this purpose.

Patient-teaching tips
• Tell patient to take medication exactly as prescribed, even if he feels better. Entire quantity prescribed should be taken.
• Tell patient to call the doctor if rash, fever, or chills develop. A rash is the most common allergic reaction.
• Warn patient never to use leftover drug for a new illness or to share it with family and friends.

Special considerations
• Before giving dicloxacillin, ask patient if he's had any allergic reactions to penicillin. However, a negative history of penicillin allergy doesn't rule out future reactions.
• Obtain specimens for culture and sensitivity tests before first dose, but don't wait for results before beginning therapy.
• Drug may cause GI upset. Food may interfere with absorption, so give drug 1 to 2 hours before meals or 2 to 3 hours after.

• With prolonged therapy, other superinfections may occur, especially in elderly or debilitated patients or those with low resistance to infection. Monitor carefully.
• Check renal, hepatic, and hematopoietic function during prolonged therapy.
• Give drug at least 1 hour before bacteriostatic antibiotics.
• Dicloxacillin appears in breast milk.

Erythromycin (E-Mycin, Erythrocin)

General
Availability: Rx.
Pregnancy risk category: B.

Classification
Pharmacologic: macrolide.
Therapeutic: antibacterial.

Pharmacokinetics
Half-life: 1½ to 2 hours (normal renal function); 5 to 6 hours (impaired renal function).
Metabolism: in various tissues, metabolized to free drug; free erythromycin then metabolized in the liver.
Excretion: in the urine and feces.

Indications and dosage
• Acute pelvic inflammatory disease caused by *Neisseria gonorrhoeae. Adults:* 500 mg (erythromycin gluceptate, lactobionate) I.V. q 6 hours for 3 days, then 250 mg (erythromycin base, estolate, stearate) or 400 mg (erythromycin ethylsuccinate) P.O. q 6 hours for 7 days.
• Endocarditis prophylaxis for dental procedures in penicillin-allergic patients. *Adults:* 1 g (erythromycin base, estolate, stearate) P.O. 1 hour before procedure, then 500 mg P.O. 6 hours later.
• Intestinal amebiasis. *Adults:* 250 mg (erythromycin base, estolate, stearate) P.O. q 6 hours for 10 to 14 days.
• Mild to moderately severe respiratory tract, skin, and soft-tissue infections caused by sensitive group A beta-hemolytic streptococci, *Diplococcus pneumoniae, Mycoplasma pneumoniae, Corynebacterium diphtheriae, Bordetella pertussis, Listeria monocytogenes. Adults:* 250 to 500 mg (erythromycin base, estolate, stearate) P.O. q 6 hours; or 400 to 800 mg (erythromycin ethylsuccinate) P.O. q 6 hours; or 15 to 20 mg/kg I.V. daily, as continuous infusion or divided q 6 hours.
• Syphilis. *Adults:* 500 mg (erythromycin base, estolate, stearate) P.O. q.i.d. for 15 days.
• Legionnaire's disease. *Adults:* 500 mg to 1 g I.V. or P.O. q 6 hours for 21 days.
• Uncomplicated urethral, endocervical, or rectal infections where tetracyclines are contraindicated. *Adults:* 500 mg P.O. q.i.d. for at least 7 days.

• Urogenital *Chlamydia trachomatis* infections during pregnancy.
Adults: 500 mg P.O. q.i.d. for at least 7 days or 250 mg P.O.
q.i.d. for at least 14 days.

Contraindications and cautions
• Erythromycin estolate contraindicated in hepatic disease.
• Use other erythromycin salts cautiously in patients with impaired hepatic function.

Adverse reactions
EENT: hearing loss with high I.V. doses.
GI: abdominal pain, cramping, nausea, vomiting, diarrhea.
Hepatic: jaundice (with erythromycin estolate).
Skin: urticaria, rash.
Local: venous irritation, thrombophlebitis after I.V. injection.
Other: overgrowth of nonsusceptible organisms, *anaphylaxis,* fever.

Interactions
Clindamycin, lincomycin: antagonistic effects.
Theophylline: decreased erythromycin blood levels and increased
theophylline toxicity. Use together cautiously.

Patient-teaching tips
• For best absorption, instruct patient to take oral form of drug
with a full glass of water 1 hour before or 2 hours after meals.
Coated tablets may be taken with meals. Tell him not to drink
fruit juice with medication and not to swallow chewable tablets
whole.
• Explain that coated forms of erythromycin cause fewer GI problems.
May be useful for patients who can't tolerate GI effects.
• Advise patient to report adverse reactions, especially nausea,
abdominal pain, or fever.

Special considerations
• Monitor hepatic function for increased levels of bilirubin, AST
(SGOT), ALT (SGPT), and alkaline phosphatase.
• Give I.V. dose over 60 minutes.
• Don't give erythromycin lactobionate with other drugs.

Gentamicin (Garamycin)

General
Availability: Rx.
Pregnancy risk category: C.

Classification
Pharmacologic: aminoglycoside.
Therapeutic: antibacterial.

Pharmacokinetics
Half-life: 2 to 3 hours (normal renal function); 40 to 50 hours
(impaired renal function).
Excretion: by kidneys, unchanged.

Indications and dosage
• Serious infections caused by sensitive *Citrobacter, Enterobacter, Escherichia coli, Klebsiella, Proteus, Pseudomonas aeruginosa, Serratia, Staphylococcus. Adults with normal renal function:* 3 mg/kg daily in divided doses q 8 hours I.M. or I.V. infusion (in 50 to 200 ml of normal saline solution or dextrose 5% in water infused over 30 minutes to 2 hours). May be given by direct I.V. push if necessary. For life-threatening infections, patient may receive up to 5 mg/kg daily in three to four divided doses. *Adults with impaired renal function:* initial dose is same as for those with normal renal function. Subsequent doses determined by renal function studies and serum drug levels.
• External eye infections. *Adults:* instill 1 to 2 drops q 4 hours. In severe infections, use up to 2 drops q 1 hour. Apply ointment to lower conjunctival sac b.i.d. or t.i.d.

Contraindications and cautions
• Contraindicated in aminoglycoside hypersensitivity.
• Use cautiously in elderly patients and in those with impaired renal function.

Adverse reactions
CNS: headache, lethargy, neuromuscular blockade.
EENT: ototoxicity (tinnitus, vertigo, hearing loss).
GU: nephrotoxicity (cells or casts in the urine; oliguria; proteinuria; decreased creatinine clearance; increased BUN, nonprotein nitrogen, and serum creatinine levels).

Interactions
Antihistamines, dimenhydrinate: possible masked symptoms of ototoxicity. Use with caution.
Cephalothin: increased nephrotoxicity. Use cautiously.
I.V. loop diuretics (such as furosemide): increased ototoxicity. Use cautiously.
Parenteral penicillins (such as carbenicillin, ticarcillin): gentamicin inactivation in vitro. Don't mix together in I.V. line.
Other aminoglycosides, methoxyflurane: increased ototoxicity and nephrotoxicity. Use together cautiously.

Patient-teaching tips
• Tell patient to notify doctor if he develops tinnitus, vertigo, or hearing loss.
• Tell patient using ocular drug to watch for symptoms of sensitivity, such as itchy lids, and to notify doctor and stop drug immediately if they occur.

Special considerations
• Obtain specimen for culture and sensitivity tests before first dose. Don't wait for results before beginning therapy.
• Weigh patient and obtain baseline renal function studies before therapy.

• Evaluate patient's hearing before and during therapy.
• Monitor renal function (urine output, specific gravity, urinalysis, BUN and creatinine levels, and creatinine clearance).
• Keep patient well hydrated while taking drug to minimize chemical irritation of the renal tubules.
• Monitor for superinfection.
• Usual duration of therapy is 7 to 10 days. If no response in 3 to 5 days, therapy may be stopped and new specimens obtained for culture and sensitivity tests.
• Peak blood levels above 12 mcg/ml and trough levels (those drawn just before next dose) above 2 mcg/ml may be associated with higher incidence of toxicity.
• Draw blood for peak gentamicin level 1 hour after I.M. injection and 30 minutes to 1 hour after infusion ends; for trough levels, draw blood just before next dose.
• Don't collect blood in a heparinized tube.
• Hemodialysis (8 hours) removes up to 50% of drug.
• If topical ocular gentamicin is given with systemic gentamicin, carefully monitor serum drug levels.

Imipenem and cilastatin (Primaxin)

General
Availability: Rx.
Pregnancy risk category: C.

Classification
Pharmacologic: combination of thienamycin derivative with renal dipeptidase inhibitor.
Therapeutic: antibacterial.

Pharmacokinetics
Half-life: 1 hour (both drugs).
Excretion: by kidneys, mostly unchanged (both drugs).

Indications and dosage
Serious infections of the lower respiratory and urinary tracts, intraabdominal and gynecologic infections, bacterial septicemia, bone and joint infections, skin and soft-tissue infections, endocarditis. Susceptible microorganisms include *Bacteroides* species, including *B. fragilis, Enterobacter* species, *Escherichia coli, Klebsiella, Proteus, Pseudomonas aeruginosa, Staphylococcus,* and *Streptococcus* species. *Adults:* 250 mg to 1 g by I.V. infusion q 6 to 8 hours. Maximum daily dosage is 50 mg/kg daily or 4 g daily, whichever is less.

Contraindications and cautions
• Use cautiously in patients allergic to penicillins or cephalosporins.
• Use cautiously in history of seizure disorders, especially if accompanied by renal impairment.

Adverse reactions
CNS: seizures, dizziness.
CV: hypotension.
GI: nausea, vomiting, diarrhea, *pseudomembranous colitis.*
Skin: rash, urticaria, pruritus.
Local: thrombophlebitis, pain at injection site.
Other: hypersensitivity.

Interactions
None significant.

Patient-teaching tips
Advise patient to tell doctor or nurse about any unusual adverse effects.

Special considerations
• Ask patient if he's had a hypersensitivity reaction to either of these drugs before administering first dose of imipenem-cilastatin. However, negative history doesn't rule out future reactions.
• Don't administer by direct I.V. bolus injection. Give each 250- or 500-mg dose by I.V. infusion over 20 to 30 minutes; each 1-g dose over 40 to 60 minutes. If nausea occurs, reduce infusion rate.
• Patients with impaired renal function may need lower dose or longer intervals between doses.
• If patient develops seizures that persist despite anticonvulsant therapy, notify doctor, then stop the drug.
• Monitor patient for bacterial or fungal superinfections and resistant infections during and after therapy.
• When reconstituting powder, shake until the solution is clear. Solutions may range from colorless to yellow, but color variations in this range don't affect potency. After reconstitution, solution is stable for 10 hours at room temperature and for 48 hours when refrigerated.
• Imipenem-cilastatin has a broad antibacterial spectrum.
It is most valuable for empiric treatment of infections and for mixed infections that would otherwise require a combination of antibiotics, in many cases including an aminoglycoside.

Nafcillin (Nafcil, Unipen)

General
Availability: Rx.
Pregnancy risk category: B.

Classification
Pharmacologic: penicillinase-resistant penicillin.
Therapeutic: antibacterial.

Pharmacokinetics
Half-life: 1¼ to 1½ hours.
Excretion: by kidneys, mainly unchanged.

Indications and dosage
Systemic infections caused by penicillinase-producing staphylococci. *Adults:* 2 to 4 g P.O. daily, divided into doses q 6 hours; 2 to 12 g I.M. or I.V. daily, divided into doses q 4 to 6 hours.

Contraindications and cautions
Use cautiously in patients with other drug allergies, especially to cephalosporins (possible cross-allergenicity), and in those with GI distress.

Adverse reactions
Blood: transient leukopenia, neutropenia, granulocytopenia, thrombocytopenia with high doses.
GI: nausea, vomiting, diarrhea.
Local: vein irritation, thrombophlebitis.
Other: hypersensitivity (chills, fever, rash, pruritus, urticaria, anaphylaxis).

Interactions
Probenecid: increased nafcillin levels. Probenecid may be used for this purpose.

Patient-teaching tips
• Instruct patient to take medication exactly as prescribed, even if he feels better. Entire quantity prescribed should be taken.
• Tell patient to call the doctor if rash, fever, or chills develop. A rash is the most common allergic reaction.

Special considerations
• Obtain specimens for culture and sensitivity tests before first dose; don't wait for test results before beginning therapy.
• Before giving nafcillin, ask patient if he's had any allergic reactions to penicillin. However, a negative history of penicillin allergy doesn't rule out a future allergic reaction.
• When given orally, drug may cause GI disturbances. Food may interfere with absorption, so give 1 to 2 hours before meals or 2 to 3 hours after.
• When giving I.V., mix with dextrose 5% in water or saline solution.
• Give I.V. intermittently to prevent vein irritation. Change site every 48 hours.
• With prolonged therapy, other superinfections may occur, especially in elderly or debilitated patients, or those with low resistance to infection from immunosuppressives or irradiation. Close observation is essential.
• Give penicillins at least 1 hour before bacteriostatic antibiotics.

Netilmicin (Netromycin)

General
Availability: Rx.
Pregnancy risk category: C.

Classification
Pharmacologic: aminoglycoside.
Therapeutic: antibacterial.

Pharmacokinetics
Half-life: 2 to 3½ hours (normal renal function); 30 hours (impaired renal function).
Excretion: by kidneys, unchanged.

Indications and dosage
Serious infections caused by sensitive *Citrobacter, Enterobacter, Escherichia coli, Klebsiella, Proteus, Pseudomonas aeruginosa, Serratia, Staphylococcus. Adults:* 3 to 6.5 mg/kg daily by I.M. injection or I.V. infusion. May be given q 12 hours to treat serious urinary tract infections and q 8 to 12 hours to treat serious systemic infections. *Patients with impaired renal function:* initial dose same as for patients with normal renal function. Subsequent doses and frequency determined by renal function studies and serum concentration of netilmicin.

Contraindications and cautions
Use cautiously in elderly patients and in those with impaired renal function.

Adverse reactions
CNS: headache, lethargy, neuromuscular blockade.
EENT: ototoxicity (tinnitus, vertigo, hearing loss).
GU: nephrotoxicity (cells or casts in the urine; oliguria; proteinuria; decreased creatinine clearance; increased BUN, nonprotein nitrogen, and serum creatinine levels).

Interactions
I.V. loop diuretics (such as furosemide): increased ototoxicity. Use cautiously.
Antihistamines, dimenhydrinate: possible masked symptoms of ototoxicity. Use with caution.
Cephalothin: increased nephrotoxicity. Use together cautiously.
Other aminoglycosides, amphotericin B, cisplatin, methoxyflurane: increased nephrotoxicity. Use together cautiously.
Parenteral penicillins (such as carbenicillin and ticarcillin): netilmicin inactivation. Don't mix together in I.V. line.

Patient-teaching tips
Urge patient to notify doctor if he develops tinnitus, vertigo, or hearing loss.

Special considerations
• Obtain specimen for culture and sensitivity tests before first dose, but don't wait for test results before beginning therapy.
• Weigh patient and obtain baseline renal function studies before therapy begins.

- Evaluate patient's hearing before and during therapy.
- Monitor renal function (urine output, specific gravity, urinalysis, BUN and creatinine levels, and creatinine clearance). Notify doctor of signs of decreasing renal function.
- Keep patient well hydrated while taking drug to minimize chemical irritation of the renal tubules.
- After completing I.V. infusion, flush the line with normal saline solution or dextrose 5% in water.
- Watch for superinfection (continued fever and other signs of new infections, especially of upper respiratory tract).
- Usual duration of therapy is 7 to 10 days. If no response in 3 to 5 days, stop therapy, as ordered, and obtain new specimens for culture and sensitivity tests.
- Peak blood levels above 16 mcg/ml and trough levels (those drawn just before next dose) above 4 mcg/ml may be associated with higher incidence of toxicity.
- Draw blood for peak netilmicin level 1 hour after I.M. injection and 30 minutes to 1 hour after infusion ends; for trough levels, draw blood just before next dose.
- Netilmicin is the newest aminoglycoside. Some studies show that this drug is less ototoxic than other drugs in its class.
- Netilmicin appears in breast milk.

Penicillin G sodium (Crystapen)

General
Availability: Rx.
Pregnancy risk category: B.

Classification
Pharmacologic: natural penicillin.
Therapeutic: antibacterial.

Pharmacokinetics
Half-life: ½ to 1 hour.
Excretion: by kidneys.

Indications and dosage
- Moderate to severe systemic infections. *Adults:* 1.2 to 24 million units daily I.M. or I.V., divided into doses given q 4 hours.
- *Endocarditis prophylaxis for dental surgery. Adults:* 2 million units I.V. or I.M. 30 to 60 minutes before procedure, then 1 million units 6 hours later.

Contraindications and cautions
- Contraindicated in patients on sodium restriction.
- Use cautiously in patients with other drug allergies, especially to cephalosporins (possible cross-allergenicity).

Adverse reactions
Blood: hemolytic anemia, leukopenia, thrombocytopenia.
CNS: arthralgia, neuropathy, convulsions.

CV: congestive heart failure with high doses.
Local: vein irritation, pain at injection site, thrombophlebitis.
Other: hypersensitivity (chills, fever, edema, maculopapular rash, exfoliative dermatitis, urticaria, anaphylaxis), overgrowth of nonsusceptible organisms.

Interactions
Probenecid: increased pencillin levels. Probenecid is often used for this purpose.

Patient-teaching tips
Tell patient to call doctor if rash, fever, or chills develop. Fever and eosinophilia are the most common allergic reactions.

Special considerations
• Obtain cultures for sensitivity tests before first dose. Unnecessary to wait for test results before beginning therapy.
• Before giving penicillin, ask patient if he's had any allergic reactions to this drug. However, a negative history of penicillin allergy is no guarantee against a future allergic reaction.
• If patient has high blood level of this drug, he may have convulsions. Be prepared by keeping side rails up on bed.
• Give I.V. intermittently to prevent vein irritation. Change site every 48 hours.
• With prolonged therapy, bacterial or fungal superinfections may occur, especially in patients who are elderly, debilitated, or who have low resistance to infection because of treatment with immunosuppressive agents or radiation.
• Give penicillins at least 1 hour before bacteriostatic antibiotics.

Tetracycline (Achromycin)
General
Availability: Rx.
Pregnancy risk category: D.

Classification
Pharmacologic: tetracycline.
Therapeutic: antibacterial.

Pharmacokinetics
Half-life: 6 to 11 hours (normal renal function); 57 to 108 hours (impaired renal function).
Excretion: in urine and feces, mainly unchanged.

Indications and dosage
• Infections caused by sensitive gram-negative and gram-positive organisms, trachoma, rickettsiae, and *Mycoplasma. Adults:* 250 to 500 mg P.O. q 6 hours; 250 mg I.M. daily or 150 mg I.M. q 12

hours; or 250 to 500 mg I.V. q 8 to 12 hours (I.M. and I.V. hydrochloride salt only).
• Uncomplicated urethral, endocervical, or rectal infection caused by *Chlamydia trachomatis. Adults:* 500 mg P.O. q.i.d. for at least 7 days.
• Gonorrhea in patients sensitive to penicillin. *Adults:* initially, 1.5 g P.O., then 500 mg q 6 hours for 7 days.
• Syphilis in patients sensitive to penicillin. *Adults:* 500 mg P.O. q.i.d. for 15 days.
• Acne. *Adults:* initially, 250 mg P.O. q 6 hours, then 125 to 500 mg P.O. daily or every other day.

Contraindications and cautions
Use with extreme caution in patients with renal or hepatic impairment.

Adverse reactions
Blood: neutropenia, eosinophilia.
CNS: dizziness, headache, intracranial hypertension.
CV: pericarditis.
EENT: sore throat, glossitis, dysphagia.
GI: anorexia, *epigastric distress, nausea,* vomiting, *diarrhea,* stomatitis, enterocolitis, inflammatory lesions in anogenital region.
Hepatic: hepatotoxicity with large doses given I.V.
Metabolic: increased BUN level.
Skin: maculopapular and erythematous rashes, urticaria, photosensitivity, increased pigmentation.
Local: irritation after I.M. injection, thrombophlebitis.

Interactions
Antacids (including NaHCO$_3$) and laxatives containing aluminum, magnesium, or calcium; food, milk, or other dairy products: decreased antibiotic absorption. Give antibiotic 1 hour before or 2 hours after.
Ferrous sulfate and other iron products, zinc: decreased antibiotic absorption. Give tetracyclines 2 hours before or 3 hours after iron administration.
Methoxyflurane: possible severe nephrotoxicity.

Patient-teaching tips
• Instruct patient to take each dose with a full glass of water on an empty stomach, at least 1 hour before meals or 2 hours afterward. Effectiveness reduced when taken with dairy products, food, antacids, or iron products.
• Warn patient to avoid direct sunlight and ultraviolet light.
• Tell patient to take medication exactly as prescribed.

Special considerations
• Obtain specimens for cultures before starting therapy.
• Patient may develop thrombophlebitis with I.V. administration.
Avoid extravasation.
• Inject I.M. dose deeply. Rotate sites. I.M. preparations often
contain local anesthetic; ask patient about allergy.
• Watch for overgrowth of nonsusceptible organisms.
• Give 1 hour before bedtime to prevent esophagitis.
• Do not mix tetracycline with any other I.V. additive.
• Parenteral form may cause false-positive urine glucose reading
with copper sulfate test (Clinitest). All forms may cause false-neg-
ative urine glucose reading with glucose oxidase test (Clinistix,
Tes-Tape).

Tobramycin (Nebcin)

General
Availability: Rx.
Pregnancy risk category: D.

Classification
Pharmacologic: aminoglycoside.
Therapeutic: antibacterial.

Pharmacokinetics
Half-life: 1.9 to 2.2 hours (normal renal function); 53 to 56 hours
(impaired renal function).
Excretion: by kidneys, unchanged.

Indications and dosage
Serious infections caused by sensitive strains of *Citrobacter, Enterobacter, Escherichia coli, Klebsiella, Proteus, Providencia,
Pseudomonas, Serratia,* and *Staphylococcus aureus. Adults with
normal renal function:* 3 mg/kg I.M. or I.V. daily divided q 8
hours. Up to 5 mg/kg I.M. or I.V. daily divided q 6 to 8 hours for
life-threatening infections. For I.V. use, dilute in 50 to 100 ml
normal saline solution or dextrose 5% in water. Infuse over 20
to 60 minutes. *Patients with impaired renal function:* initial
dose same as for patients with normal renal function. Subsequent dosage determined by results of renal function studies and
serum levels of tobramycin.

Contraindications and cautions
Use cautiously in patients with renal impairment and in elderly
patients.

Adverse reactions
CNS: headache, lethargy, *neuromuscular blockade.*
EENT: ototoxicity (tinnitus, vertigo, hearing loss).
*GU: nephrotoxicity (cells or casts in urine, oliguria, proteinuria,
decreased creatinine clearance, increased BUN and serum cre-
atinine levels).*

Interactions

Amphotericin B, cisplatin, methoxyflurane, other aminoglycosides: increased ototoxicity and nephrotoxicity. Use together cautiously.
Cephalothin: increased nephrotoxicity. Use together cautiously.
Dimenhydrinate: possibly masked symptoms of ototoxicity. Use cautiously.
I.V. loop diuretics (such as furosemide): increased ototoxicity. Use cautiously.
Parenteral penicillins (such as carbenicillin and ticarcillin): tobramycin inactivation in vitro. Don't mix together in I.V. line.

Patient-teaching tips

• Instruct patient to notify doctor if he develops tinnitus, vertigo, or hearing loss.
• Tell female patient to notify doctor if she becomes pregnant while taking this drug.

Special considerations

• Obtain specimen for culture and sensitivity tests before first dose, but don't wait for test results before beginning therapy.
• Weigh patient and obtain baseline renal function studies before starting therapy.
• Evaluate patient's hearing before and during therapy.
• Usual duration of therapy is 7 to 10 days.
• Monitor renal function. Notify doctor of signs of decreasing renal function.
• Patient should be well hydrated while taking drug to minimize chemical irritation of renal tubules.
• Watch for superinfection (continued fever and other signs of new infections, especially of upper respiratory tract).
• Peak blood levels over 12 mcg/ml and trough levels above 2 mcg/ml may be associated with increased incidence of toxicity.
• Draw blood for peak tobramycin level 1 hour after I.M. injection and 30 minutes to 1 hour after infusion ends; draw blood for trough level just before next dose.
• Don't collect blood in a heparinized tube.
• After I.V. infusion, flush line with normal saline solution or dextrose 5% in water.
• Studies indicate tobramycin is less nephrotoxic than gentamicin.

Vancomycin (Vancocin)

General

Availability: Rx.
Pregnancy risk category: C.

Classification

Pharmacologic: glycopeptide.
Therapeutic: antibacterial.

Pharmacokinetics
Half-life: 6 hours (normal renal function); 6 to 10 days (impaired renal function).
Metabolism: mainly in liver.
Excretion: by kidneys.

Indications and dosage
• Severe staphylococcal infections when other antibiotics ineffective or contraindicated. *Adults:* 500 mg I.V. q 6 hours, or 1 g q 12 hours.
• Antibiotic-associated pseudomembranous and staphylococcal enterocolitis. *Adults:* 125 to 500 mg P.O. q 6 hours for 7 to 10 days.
• Endocarditis prophylaxis for dental procedures. *Adults:* 1 g I.V. slowly over 1 hour, starting 1 hour before procedure. No repeat dose is necessary.

Contraindications and cautions
Use cautiously in patients receiving other neurotoxic, nephrotoxic, or ototoxic drugs; in those with hepatic or renal impairment; in those with preexisting hearing loss; in patients over 60 years; and in patients with allergies to other antibiotics.

Adverse reactions
Blood: transient eosinophilia, leukopenia.
EENT: tinnitus, ototoxicity (deafness).
GI: nausea.
Skin: "red-neck" syndrome (maculopapular rash on face, neck, trunk, or extremities).
Local: pain or thrombophlebitis with I.V. administration, necrosis.
Other: chills, fever, *anaphylaxis,* overgrowth of nonsusceptible organisms.

Interactions
None significant.

Patient-teaching tips
• Instruct patient to take medication exactly as directed, even after he feels better.
• Warn patient to report adverse reactions at once, especially fullness or ringing in ears. He should stop drug immediately if these occur.

Special considerations
• Patients should receive auditory function tests before and during prolonged therapy.
• Monitor renal function (BUN and serum creatinine levels, urinalysis, creatinine clearance, urine output) before and during therapy. Watch for signs of superinfection.
• Monitor patient carefully for "red-neck" syndrome. Stop infusion and notify doctor if you see this reaction.
• Patients with renal dysfunction may require adjusted dosage.
• Do not give drug I.M.

• For I.V. infusion, dilute in 200 ml sodium chloride injection or 5% glucose solution. Check site daily for phlebitis and irritation. Report pain at infusion site. Avoid extravasation. Severe irritation and necrosis can result.
• Refrigerate I.V. solution after reconstitution and use within 4 days.
• Oral preparation stable for 2 weeks if refrigerated.

☐ Preoperative medications

Preoperative medications are used to relieve anxiety, provide sedation, induce amnesia, decrease salivation and gastric secretions, elevate gastric pH, and prevent allergic reactions to anesthetic agents. Such medications usually are administered 1 to 2 hours before induction of anesthesia.

Below is a list of some of the most commonly prescribed preoperative medications. (*Note:* Italicized adverse reactions are common or life-threatening.)

Atropine

General
Availability: Rx (non-Rx in Canada).
Pregnancy risk category: C.

Classification
Pharmacologic: anticholinergic.
Therapeutic: antiarrhythmic, antispasmodic.

Pharmacokinetics
Half-life: 13 to 38 hours.
Onset: 30 minutes (diminished secretions); 5 minutes (increased heart rate).
Peak: 1½ to 2 hours (diminished secretions); 20 to 60 minutes (increased heart rate).
Metabolism: partly in liver.
Excretion: by kidneys as unchanged and metabolized drug.

Indications and dosage
• Adjunctive therapy in peptic ulcers, irritable bowel syndrome, neurogenic bowel disturbances, and functional GI disorders. *Adults:* 0.25 to 0.6 mg P.O. q 4 to 6 hours.
• Symptomatic bradycardia, bradydysrhythmia (junctional or escape rhythm). *Adults:* usually 0.5 to 1 mg I.V. push; repeat q 5 minutes, to maximum 2 mg. Lower doses (less than 0.5 mg) can cause bradycardia.
• Antidote for anticholinesterase insecticide poisoning. *Adults:* 2 mg I.M. or I.V. repeated at hourly intervals until muscarinic symptoms disappear. Severe cases may require up to 6 mg I.M. or I.V. q 1 hour.

• Preoperative reduction of secretions and blockage of cardiac vagal reflexes. *Adults:* 0.4 to 0.6 mg I.M. 45 to 60 minutes before anesthesia.

Contraindications and cautions

Contraindicated in narrow-angle glaucoma, obstructive uropathy, obstructive GI disease, myasthenia gravis, paralytic ileus, intestinal atony, unstable cardiovascular status in acute hemorrhage, and toxic megacolon.

Adverse reactions

Blood: leukocytosis.
CNS: headache, restlessness, ataxia, disorientation, hallucinations, delirium, coma, *insomnia, dizziness,* excitement, agitation, and confusion (especially in elderly patients).
CV: 1 to 2 mg—*tachycardia, palpitations;* greater than 2 mg—*extreme tachycardia, angina.*
EENT: 1 mg—*slight mydriasis,* photophobia; 2 mg—*blurred vision, mydriasis.*
GI: dry mouth (common even at low doses), thirst, *constipation, nausea, vomiting.*
GU: urine retention.
Skin: hot, flushed skin.

Interactions

Methotrimeprazine: possible extrapyramidal symptoms.
Other anticholinergics: increased vagal blockage.

Patient-teaching tips

• Instruct patient to avoid driving and other hazardous activities if he is drowsy, dizzy, or has blurred vision; to drink plenty of fluids to help prevent constipation; and to report any skin rash.
• Suggest using gum, sugarless hard candy, or pilocarpine syrup to relieve mouth dryness. Saliva substitute may be necessary.

Special considerations

• *Treatment for overdose:* Antimuscarinic symptoms, such as blurred vision, require physostigmine.
• Give 30 minutes to 1 hour before meals and at bedtime. Bedtime dose can be larger and should be given at least 2 hours after last meal of day.
• Adverse reactions are dose-related and expected.
• Watch for tachycardia in cardiac patients.
• When given I.V., drug may cause paradoxical initial bradycardia. Usually disappears within 2 minutes.
• Monitor intake and output. Drug causes urine retention and hesitancy; have patient void before receiving the drug.
• Monitor closely for urine retention in elderly males with benign prostatic hypertrophy.
• Atropine also given as an ophthalmic solution in treating acute iris inflammation and cycloplegic refraction.

Diazepam (Valium)

General
Availability: Rx.
Pregnancy risk category: D.
Controlled substance schedule: IV.

Classification
Pharmacologic: benzodiazepine.
Therapeutic: antianxiety agent, sedative-hypnotic, anticonvulsant.

Pharmacokinetics
Half-life: 20 to 70 hours.
Onset: 15 to 45 minutes (P.O.); 20 minutes (I.M.); 1 to 3 minutes (I.V.).
Metabolism: in liver.
Excretion: by kidneys as metabolites.

Indications and dosage
• Tension, anxiety, adjunct in convulsive disorders or skeletal muscle spasm. *Adults:* 2 to 10 mg P.O. t.i.d. or q.i.d. Or 15 to 30 mg of extended-release capsule once daily.
• Tension, anxiety, muscle spasm, endoscopic procedures, seizures. *Adults:* 5 to 10 mg I.V. initially, up to 30 mg in 1 hour or more for cardioversion, depending on response.
• Status epilepticus. *Adults:* 5 to 20 mg slow I.V. push 2 to 5 mg/minute; may repeat q 5 to 10 minutes up to maximum total dosage of 60 mg. Use 2 to 5 mg in elderly or debilitated patients. May repeat in 20 to 30 minutes with caution if seizures recur.
• Preoperative sedation. *Adults:* 5 to 15 mg P.O.

Contraindications and cautions
• Contraindicated in shock, coma, acute alcohol intoxication, acute narrow-angle glaucoma, psychoses, and myasthenia gravis.
• Use cautiously in patients with blood dyscrasias, hepatic or renal damage, depression, open-angle glaucoma; in elderly and debilitated patients; and in those with limited pulmonary reserve.

Adverse reactions
CNS: drowsiness, lethargy, hangover, ataxia, fainting, slurred speech, tremors.
CV: transient hypotension, bradycardia, *cardiovascular collapse.*
EENT: diplopia, blurred vision, nystagmus.
GI: nausea, vomiting, abdominal discomfort.
Skin: rash, urticaria.
Local: desquamation, *pain, phlebitis at injection site.*
Other: respiratory depression.

Interactions
Alcohol, CNS depressants: increased CNS depression. Avoid concomitant use.
Cimetidine: increased sedation. Monitor carefully.

Phenobarbital: increased effects of both drugs. Use together cautiously.

Patient-teaching tips
• Tell patient to avoid activities requiring alertness and psychomotor coordination.
• Warn him not to use alcohol or other depressants.
• Caution patient against giving medication to others.
• Tell female patient to notify doctor if she becomes pregnant while taking this drug.

Special considerations
• *Treatment for overdose:* For hypotension, give vasopressors.
• Monitor respirations every 5 to 15 minutes and before each I.V. dose. Have resuscitation equipment and oxygen nearby. Naloxone doesn't reverse respiratory depression.
• Possibility of abuse and addiction exists. Don't withdraw drug abruptly; withdrawal symptoms may occur.
• Incompatible with all solutions and drugs. Don't store diazepam in plastic syringes.
• Avoid extravasation. Don't inject into small veins.
• Give I.V. slowly, not exceeding 5 mg/minute. When injecting I.V., administer directly into the vein.
• I.V. route is more reliable; I.M. absorption is variable. I.M. administration is also painful.
• Drug of choice (I.V. form) for status epilepticus.
• Not to be prescribed regularly for everyday stress.

Hydroxyzine (Atarax, Vistaril)

General
Availability: Rx.
Pregnancy risk category: C.

Classification
Pharmacologic: antihistamine (piperazine derivative).
Therapeutic: antianxiety agent.

Pharmacokinetics
Onset: 15 to 30 minutes.
Duration: 4 to 6 hours.
Metabolism: in liver.
Excretion: by kidneys.

Indications and dosage
• Anxiety and tension. *Adults:* 25 to 100 mg P.O. t.i.d. or q.i.d.
• Preoperative and postoperative adjunctive therapy. *Adults:* 25 to 100 mg I.M. q 4 to 6 hours.

Contraindications and cautions
Contraindicated in shock or coma.

Adverse reactions
CNS: drowsiness, involuntary motor activity.
GI: dry mouth.
Local: pain at I.M. injection site.

Interactions
Alcohol, CNS depressants: increased CNS depression. Avoid concomitant use.

Patient-teaching tips
• Warn patient to avoid activities requiring alertness and good psychomotor coordination until CNS response to drug is determined.
• Warn him not to combine drug with alcohol or other CNS depressants.
• Suggest to the patient that sugarless hard candy or gum relieves dry mouth.

Special considerations
• *Treatment for overdose:* In hypotension, give vasopressors (but *not* epinephrine); in CNS depression, give caffeine sodium benzoate injection.
• Monitor for excessive sedation from potentiation with other CNS drugs.
• Parenteral form (hydroxyzine HCl) for I.M. use only, never I.V. Use Z-track injection.
• Aspirate injection carefully to prevent inadvertent intravascular injection. Inject deep into a large muscle.
• Used as an antiemetic and antianxiety drug.
• Used in psychogenically induced allergic conditions, such as chronic urticaria and pruritus.
• Reduce dosage in elderly or debilitated patients.

Midazolam (Versed)

General
Availability: Rx.
Pregnancy risk category: D.
Controlled substance schedule: IV.

Classification
Pharmacologic: benzodiazepine.
Therapeutic: sedative.

Pharmacokinetics
Half-life: 1¾ to 4 hours.
Onset: 15 minutes (I.M.).
Peak: 30 to 60 minutes (I.M.).
Metabolism: in liver.
Excretion: by kidneys.

Indications and dosage

• Preoperative sedation (to induce sleepiness or drowiness and relieve apprehension). *Adults:* 0.07 mg to 0.08 mg/kg I.M. approximately 1 hour before surgery. May be administered with atropine or scopolamine and reduced doses of narcotics.

• Conscious sedation before short diagnostic or endoscopic procedures. *Adults:* initially, 0.035 mg/kg slow I.V., then titrated in small amounts to a total dosage of 0.1 mg/kg. Do not exceed 2.5 mg in normal healthy adults; lower doses indicated in elderly or debilitated patients, and in those receiving narcotics concomitantly.

• Induction of general anesthesia. *Adults:* 0.3 to 0.35 mg/kg I.V. over 20 to 30 seconds. Additional increments of 25% of the initial dose may be needed to complete induction. Total dosage up to 0.6 mg/kg.

Contraindications and cautions

• Contraindicated in patients with acute narrow-angle glaucoma.

• Don't give to patients in shock, coma, or acute alcohol intoxication.

Adverse reactions

CNS: headache, oversedation.
CV: variations in blood pressure and pulse rate.
GI: nausea, vomiting, hiccups.
Local: pain and tenderness at injection site.
Other: decreased respiratory rate, apnea.

Interactions

CNS depressants: possible increased risk of apnea. Prepare to adjust drug dosage.

Patient-teaching tips

• Advise patient to postpone tasks that require mental alertness or physical coordination until the drug's effects have worn off.

• As necessary, instruct patient in safety measures, such as supervised ambulation and gradual position changes, to prevent injury.

• Advise patient to notify doctor if he is taking any nonprescription drugs.

Special considerations

• Before administering midazolam I.V., have oxygen and resuscitative equipment available in case of severe respiratory depression. Excessive dosage or rapid infusion has been associated with respiratory arrest, especially in elderly or debilitated patients.

• Monitor blood pressure during procedure, especially in patients who have also been premedicated with narcotics.

• When injecting I.M., give deep into a large muscle mass.

• When administering I.V., take care to avoid extravasation.

• May be mixed in the same syringe with morphine sulfate, meperidine, atropine sulfate, or scopolamine.

• Midazolam has a beneficial amnesic effect, which diminishes patient's recall of perioperative events. This drug offers advantages over diazepam, hydroxyzine, and barbiturates, which are prescribed for similar indications.

☐ Analgesics

Analgesics are used postoperatively to control pain. Narcotics, the most common type of analgesics administered, may be given I.M. or I.V. Because the dosage needed to achieve effective pain control varies from patient to patient (and even varies from time to time within the same patient), you'll need to observe each patient closely for evidence of desired effectiveness.

Narcotics can become addictive; however, when used solely to treat postoperative pain (usually for 7 to 10 days), drug addiction rarely occurs. Other nonnarcotic analgesics, such as propoxyphene and acetaminophen, usually are given after the first few postoperative days for patients who continue to experience discomfort.

Self-administered, or "on-demand," analgesia has recently been used to treat postoperative pain. This new administration method improves pain control and lowers the total dosage of analgesic given over a 24-hour period. With this method, a patient in pain depresses a button at his bedside that triggers an infusion pump with a timing unit. A predetermined dose of analgesic (usually 1 to 1.5 mg of morphine) is delivered via the patient's I.V. line.

To prevent overdosage with self-administration, the dosage and timing are programmed, as ordered, into the infusion mechanism to accommodate the patient's needs. As a special precaution, the mechanism is programmed for periods of inactivation, during which time medication cannot be dispensed.

Below is a list of analgesics commonly prescribed during the postoperative period. (*Note:* Italicized adverse reactions are common or life-threatening.)

Codeine

General
Availability: Rx.
Pregnancy risk category: C (D if in prolonged therapy or in high doses at term).
Controlled substance schedule: II.

Classification
Pharmacologic: opiate agonist.
Therapeutic: antitussive, narcotic analgesic.

Pharmacokinetics
Onset: 10 to 30 minutes (I.M. or S.C.); 30 to 45 minutes (P.O.).
Peak: 30 to 60 minutes (I.M. or S.C.); 60 to 120 minutes (P.O.).
Duration: 4 hours (all forms). *Note:* Antitussive action may last slightly longer.
Metabolism: in liver to active and inactive metabolites.
Excretion: by kidneys, partially as unchanged drug.

Indications and dosage
• Mild to moderate pain. *Adults:* 15 to 60 mg P.O. or 15 to 60 mg (phosphate) S.C. or I.M. q 4 hours, p.r.n. or around the clock.
• Nonproductive cough. *Adults:* 8 to 20 mg P.O. q 4 to 6 hours. Maximum 120 mg/24 hours.

Contraindications and cautions
• Use with extreme caution in patients with head injury, increased intracranial pressure (ICP), hepatic or renal disease, hypothyroidism, Addison's disease, acute alcoholism, seizures, severe CNS depression, bronchial asthma, chronic obstructive pulmonary disease (COPD), respiratory depression, or shock.
• Also use with extreme caution in elderly or debilitated patients.

Adverse reactions
CNS: sedation, clouded sensorium, euphoria, seizures with large doses, dizziness.
CV: hypotension, bradycardia.
GI: nausea, vomiting, constipation, dry mouth, ileus.
GU: urine retention.
Skin: pruritus, flushing.
Other: respiratory depression, physical dependence.

Interactions
Other CNS depressants (alcohol, general anesthetics, hypnotics, monoamine oxidase [MAO] inhibitors, other narcotic analgesics, sedatives, tranquilizers, tricyclic antidepressants): additive effects. Use together cautiously. Monitor patient response.

Patient-teaching tips
Warn ambulatory patient to avoid activities that require alertness.

Special considerations
• *Treatment for overdose:* For respiratory depression, administer naloxone.
• Monitor respiratory and circulatory status and bowel function.
• For full analgesic effect, give before patient has intense pain.
• Codeine and aspirin or acetaminophen are often prescribed together to provide enhanced pain relief.
• Don't administer discolored injection solution.
• An antitussive; don't use when cough is a valuable diagnostic sign or beneficial (as after thoracic surgery).
• Monitor cough type and frequency.
• Constipating effect makes codeine useful for treating diarrhea.

Hydromorphone (Dilaudid)

General
Availability: Rx.
Pregnancy risk category: B (D if used for prolonged periods or in high doses).
Controlled substance schedule: II.

Classification
Pharmacologic: opiate agonist.
Therapeutic: narcotic analgesic, antitussive.

Pharmacokinetics
Onset: 30 minutes (P.O.); 15 minutes (I.M.); 10 to 15 minutes (I.V.); 15 minutes (S.C.).
Peak: 30 to 50 minutes (P.O., I.M., or S.C.); 15 to 30 minutes (I.V.).
Duration: 4 hours (P.O., I.M., or S.C.); 2 to 3 hours (I.V.).
Metabolism: in liver.
Excretion: by kidneys.

Indications and dosage
• Moderate to severe pain. *Adults:* 1 to 6 mg P.O. q 4 to 6 hours, p.r.n. or around the clock; or 2 to 4 mg I.M., S.C., or I.V. q 4 to 6 hours, p.r.n. or around the clock (I.V. dose should be given over 3 to 5 minutes); or 3 mg rectal suppository at bedtime, p.r.n. or q 6 to 8 hours around the clock.
• Cough. *Adults:* 1 mg P.O. q 3 to 4 hours, p.r.n.

Contraindications and cautions
• Contraindicated in increased ICP and status asthmaticus.
• Use with extreme caution in patients with increased CSF pressure, respiratory depression, hepatic or renal disease, hypothyroidism, shock, Addison's disease, acute alcoholism, seizures, head injury, severe CNS depression, brain tumor, bronchial asthma, COPD, and in elderly or debilitated patients.

Adverse reactions
CNS: sedation, somnolence, clouded sensorium, euphoria, convulsions with large doses.
CV: hypotension, bradycardia.
GI: nausea, vomiting, constipation, ileus.
GU: urine retention.
Local: induration with repeated S.C. injection.
Other: respiratory depression, physical dependence.

Interactions
Alcohol, CNS depressants: additive effects. Use together cautiously.

Patient-teaching tips
• Warn ambulatory patient to avoid activities that require alertness.
• When used postoperatively, encourage patient to turn, cough, and deep-breathe to avoid atelectasis.

Special considerations
• *Treatment for overdose:* In respiratory depression, give naloxone.
• Keep narcotic antagonist (naloxone) available.
• Respiratory depression and hypotension can occur with I.V. administration. Give slowly and monitor vital signs constantly. Also monitor bowel function.
• Rotate injection sites.
• Commonly abused narcotic. Considered more addictive than codeine.
• Oral dosage form is particularly convenient for patients with chronic pain.
• For better analgesic effect, give before patient has intense pain.
• Cough syrup is an antitussive; don't use when cough is valuable diagnostic sign or beneficial (as after thoracic surgery).
• Monitor cough type and frequency.

Meperidine (Demerol)

General
Availability: Rx.
Pregnancy risk category: B (D if used for prolonged periods or in high doses at term).
Controlled substance schedule: II.

Classification
Pharmacologic: opiate agonist.
Therapeutic: narcotic analgesic.

Pharmacokinetics
Onset: 15 minutes (P.O.); 10 to 15 minutes (I.M. or S.C.); 1 minute (I.V.).
Peak: 60 to 90 minutes (P.O.); 30 to 50 minutes (I.M. or S.C.); 5 to 7 minutes (I.V.).
Duration: 2 to 4 hours (all forms).
Metabolism: in liver to active and inactive metabolites.
Excretion: by kidneys.

Indications and dosage
• Moderate to severe pain. *Adults:* 50 to 150 mg P.O., I.M., or S.C. q 3 to 4 hours, p.r.n. or around the clock.
• Preoperative medication. *Adults:* 50 to 100 mg I.M. or S.C. 30 to 90 minutes before surgery.

Contraindications and cautions
• Contraindicated if patient has used MAO inhibitors within 14 days.
• Use with extreme caution in patients with increased ICP, shock, CNS depression, head injury, asthma, COPD, respiratory depression, supraventricular tachycardias, seizures, acute abdominal conditions, hepatic or renal disease, hypothyroidism, Addison's disease, urethral stricture, prostatic hypertrophy, or alcoholism; and in elderly or debilitated patients.

Adverse reactions
CNS: sedation, somnolence, clouded sensorium, euphoria, convulsions with large doses, paradoxical excitement, tremors.
CV: hypotension, bradycardia, tachycardia.
GI: nausea, vomiting, constipation, ileus.
GU: urine retention.
Local: pain at injection site, local tissue irritation and induration after S.C. injection; phlebitis after I.V. injection.
Other: respiratory depression, physical dependence, muscle twitching.

Interactions
Alcohol, CNS depressants: additive effects. Use together cautiously.
Barbiturates, isoniazid, MAO inhibitors: increased CNS excitation or depression; can be severe or fatal. Don't use together.
Phenytoin: decreased blood levels of meperidine. Monitor for decreased analgesia.

Patient-teaching tips
• Warn ambulatory patient to avoid activities requiring alertness until CNS response to drug is determined.
• When used postoperatively, encourage patient to turn, cough, and deep-breathe to avoid atelectasis.

Special considerations
• *Treatment for overdose:* In respiratory depression, give naloxone.
• Keep naloxone available when giving drug I.V.
• Meperidine and active metabolite normeperidine accumulate. Monitor for increased toxic effect, especially in patients with poor renal function.
• Monitor respiratory and cardiovascular status carefully. Don't give if respirations are below 12/minute or if change in pupils is noted.
• For better analgesic effect, give before patient has intense pain.
• Oral dose less than half as effective as parenteral dose. Give I.M. if possible. When changing from parenteral to oral route, dose should be increased.
• May be given slow I.V., preferably as a diluted solution. S.C. injection is very painful.
• Syrup has local anesthetic effect. Give with full glass of water.
• Watch for withdrawal symptoms if stopped abruptly after long-term use.
• May be used in some patients allergic to morphine.

Morphine

General
Availability: Rx.
Pregnancy risk category: B (D if used for prolonged periods or in high doses at term).
Controlled substance schedule: II.

Classification
Pharmacologic: opiate agonist.
Therapeutic: narcotic analgesic.

Pharmacokinetics
Onset: 10 to 30 minutes (P.O., I.M., or S.C.); 20 to 60 minutes (rectal); 5 minutes (I.V.).
Peak: 60 to 90 minutes (P.O., I.M., or S.C.); 20 minutes (I.V.).
Duration: 4 to 5 minutes (P.O., I.V., I.M., or S.C.); 8 to 12 minutes (extended-release P.O.).
Metabolism: mainly in liver.
Excretion: mainly by kidneys.

Indications and dosage
Severe pain. *Adults:* 4 to 15 mg S.C. or I.M., or 30 to 60 mg P.O. or by rectum q 4 hours, p.r.n. or around the clock. May be injected slow I.V. (over 4 to 5 minutes) diluted in 4 to 5 ml water for injection. May also administer controlled-release tablets q 8 to 12 hours. As an epidural injection, 5 mg via an epidural catheter q 24 hours. In some situations, morphine may be administered by continuous I.V. infusion or by intraspinal and intrathecal injection.

Contraindications and cautions
Use with extreme caution in patients with head injury, increased ICP, seizures, asthma, COPD, alcoholism, prostatic hypertrophy, severe hepatic or renal disease, acute abdominal conditions, hypothyroidism, Addison's disease, urethral stricture, dysrhythmias, reduced blood volume, or toxic psychosis; and in elderly or debilitated patients.

Adverse reactions
CNS: sedation, somnolence, clouded sensorium, euphoria, convulsions with large doses, *nightmares* (with long-acting forms).
CV: hypotension, bradycardia.
GI: nausea, vomiting, constipation, ileus.
GU: urine retention.
Other: respiratory depression, physical dependence, pruritus and skin flushing (with epidural administration).

Interactions
Alcohol, CNS depressants: possible additive effects. Monitor patient response.

MAO inhibitors, tricyclic antidepressants: possible respiratory depression, hypotension, profound sedation, or coma. Avoid giving concomitantly.

Patient-teaching tips
• Warn ambulatory patient to avoid activities requiring alertness until CNS response to drug has been determined.
• Tell patient that constipation is often severe with maintenance. Make sure stool softener or other laxative is ordered.
• When used postoperatively, encourage patient to turn, cough, and deep-breathe to avoid atelectasis.

Special considerations
• *Treatment for overdose:* In respiratory depression, give naloxone.
• Keep narcotic antagonist (naloxone) and resuscitative equipment available.
• Monitor circulatory and respiratory status and bowel function. Don't give if respirations are below 12/minute.
• Oral solutions of various concentrations are available. Be sure to note the strength you are administering.
• Sublingual administration may be ordered. Measure out oral solution with tuberculin syringe. Administer dose a few drops at a time to allow maximal sublingual absorption and to minimize swallowing.
• Preservative-free preparations now available for epidural and intrathecal administration. Epidural route is increasingly popular.
• When given epidurally, monitor closely for respiratory depression up to 24 hours after the epidural injection. Check respiratory rate and depth every 30 to 60 minutes for 24 hours.
• May worsen or mask gallbladder pain.
• Morphine appears in breast milk.

Oxycodone (Roxicodone)

General
Availability: Rx.
Pregnancy risk category: B (D if used for prolonged periods or in high doses at term).
Controlled substance schedule: II.

Classification
Pharmacologic: opiate agonist.
Therapeutic: narcotic analgesic.

Pharmacokinetics
Onset: 10 to 15 minutes.
Peak: 60 minutes.
Duration: 3 to 4 hours.
Metabolism: in liver.
Excretion: by kidneys.

Indications and dosage
Moderate to severe pain. *Adults:* 5 mg oxycodone P.O. q 6 hours. Or one to three suppositories (Supeudol) given rectally daily, p.r.n. or around the clock. Or in combination with other drugs, such as aspirin (Percodan, Percodan-Demi), or acetaminophen (Percocet, Tylox), one to two tablets P.O. q 6 hours, p.r.n. or around the clock.

Contraindications and cautions
Use with extreme caution in patients with head injury, increased ICP, increased CSF pressure, seizures, asthma, COPD, alcoholism, prostatic hypertrophy, severe hepatic or renal disease, acute abdominal conditions, urethral stricture, hypothyroidism, Addison's disease, dysrhythmias, reduced blood volume, toxic psychosis, and in elderly or debilitated patients.

Adverse reactions
CNS: sedation, somnolence, clouded sensorium, euphoria, convulsions with large doses.
CV: hypotension, bradycardia.
GI: nausea, vomiting, constipation, ileus.
GU: urine retention.
Other: respiratory depression, physical dependence.

Interactions
Alcohol, CNS depressants, MAO inhibitors, tricyclic antidepressants: increased CNS depression. Use together cautiously.
Anticoagulants: with oxycodone hydrochloride products containing aspirin, possible increased anticoagulant effect. Monitor clotting times. Use together cautiously.

Patient-teaching tips
Warn ambulatory patient to avoid activities requiring alertness.

Special considerations
• *Treatment for overdose:* For respiratory depression, give naloxone.
• Monitor circulatory and respiratory status and bowel function. Do not give if respirations are below 12/minute.
• For full analgesic effect, give before patient has intense pain.
• Give after meals or with milk.
• Single-agent oxycodone solution or tablets are especially good for patients who shouldn't take aspirin or acetaminophen.
• Has high abuse potential.

Appendix: NANDA Taxonomy of Nursing Diagnoses

A taxonomy for discussing nursing diagnoses has evolved over several years. The following list contains the approved diagnostic labels of the North American Nursing Diagnosis Association, as of summer 1988.

Activity intolerance
Activity intolerance: Potential
Adjustment, impaired
Airway clearance, ineffective
Anxiety
Aspiration, potential for
Body temperature, altered: Potential
Bowel elimination, altered: Colonic constipation
Bowel elimination, altered: Constipation
Bowel elimination, altered: Diarrhea
Bowel elimination, altered: Incontinence
Bowel elimination, altered: Perceived constipation
Breast-feeding, ineffective
Breathing pattern, ineffective
Cardiac output, altered: Decreased
Comfort, altered: Pain
Comfort, altered: Chronic pain
Communication, impaired: Verbal
Coping, family: Potential for growth
Coping, ineffective: Defensive
Coping, ineffective: Denial
Coping, ineffective family: Compromised
Coping, ineffective family: Disabled
Coping, ineffective individual
Decisional conflict (specify)
Disuse syndrome, potential for
Diversional activity, deficit
Dysreflexia
Family processes, altered
Fatigue
Fear
Fluid volume deficit: Actual (1)
Fluid volume deficit: Actual (2)
Fluid volume deficit: Potential
Fluid volume excess
Gas exchange, impaired
Grieving, anticipatory
Grieving, dysfunctional
Growth and development, altered
Health maintenance, altered
Health-seeking behaviors (specify)
Home maintenance management, impaired
Hopelessness
Hyperthermia
Hypothermia
Incontinence, functional

Incontinence, reflex
Incontinence, stress
Incontinence, total
Incontinence, urge
Infection, potential for
Injury, potential for
Injury, potential for: Poisoning
Injury, potential for: Suffocating
Injury, potential for: Trauma
Knowledge deficit (specify)
Mobility, impaired physical
Noncompliance (specify)
Nutrition, altered: Less than body requirements
Nutrition, altered: More than body requirements
Nutrition, altered: Potential for more than body requirements
Parental role, conflict
Parenting, altered: Actual
Parenting, altered: Potential
Post-trauma response
Powerlessness
Rape-trauma syndrome
Rape-trauma syndrome: Compound reaction
Rape-trauma syndrome: Silent reaction
Role performance, altered
Self-care deficit: Bathing/hygiene
Self-care deficit: Dressing/grooming
Self-care deficit: Feeding
Self-care deficit: Toileting
Self-concept, disturbance in: Body image
Self-concept, disturbance in: Personal identity
Self-esteem, chronic low
Self-esteem, disturbance in
Self-esteem, situational low
Sensory-perceptual alteration: Visual, auditory, kinesthetic, gustatory,
   tactile, olfactory
Sexual dysfunction
Sexuality, altered patterns
Skin integrity, impaired: Actual
Skin integrity, impaired: Potential
Sleep pattern disturbance
Social interaction, impaired
Social isolation
Spiritual distress (distress of the human spirit)
Swallowing, impaired
Thermoregulation, ineffective
Thought processes, altered
Tissue integrity, impaired
Tissue integrity, impaired: Oral mucous membrane
Tissue perfusion, altered: Renal, cerebral, cardiopulmonary,
   gastrointestinal, peripheral
Unilateral neglect
Urinary elimination, altered patterns
Urine retention
Violence, potential for: Self-directed or directed at others

Selected References

Books

Bates, B. *A Guide to Physical Examination,* 3rd ed. Philadelphia: J.B. Lippincott Co., 1983.

Beare, P.G., et al. *Nursing Implications of Diagnostic Tests,* 2nd ed. Philadelphia: J.B. Lippincott Co., 1985.

Bowers, A.C., and Thompson, J.M. *Clinical Manual of Health Assessment,* 2nd ed. St. Louis: C.V. Mosby Co., 1984.

Brunner, L.S., and Suddarth, D.S. *Textbook of Medical-Surgical Nursing,* 5th ed. Philadelphia: J.B. Lippincott Co., 1984.

Carpenito, L.J. *Nursing Diagnosis: Application to Clinical Practice.* Philadelphia: J.B. Lippincott Co., 1983.

Emergencies. Nurse's Reference Library. Springhouse, Pa.: Springhouse Corp., 1985.

Guyton, A.C. *Textbook of Medical Physiology,* 7th ed. Philadelphia: W.B. Saunders Co., 1986.

Malasanos, L. *Health Assessment,* 2nd ed. St. Louis: C.V. Mosby Co., 1981.

Michaels, D., ed. *Diagnostic Procedures: The Patient and the Health Care Team.* New York: John Wiley & Sons, 1983.

Sodeman, W.A., and Sodeman, T.M. *Pathologic Physiology: Mechanisms of Disease,* 7th ed. Philadelphia: W.B. Saunders Co., 1985.

Way, W.L., ed. *Current Surgical Diagnosis and Treatment,* 7th ed. Los Altos, Calif.: Lange Medical Pub., 1985.

Periodicals

Cass, A.C. "The Multiple Injured Patient with Bladder Trauma," *Journal of Trauma* 24(8):731-34, August 1984.

Frame, P.T. "Acute Infectious Pneumonia in the Adult," *Respiratory Care* 28(1):100-09, January 1983.

MacLaren, I.F. "Recognition and Management of Abdominal Injuries," *Surgery Annals* 14:181-219, 1982.

Rice, V. "Shock Management, Part I: Fluid Volume Replacement," *Critical Care Nurse* 4(6):69-82, November/December 1984.

Rice, V. "Shock Management, Part II: Pharmacologic Intervention," *Critical Care Nurse* 5(1):42-57, January/February 1985.

Sharma, G.V., et al. "Clinical and Hemodynamic Correlates in Pulmonary Embolism," *Clinical Chest Medicine* 5(3):421-37, September 1984.

Walker, S. "Understanding X-ray Films," *Journal of Emergency Nursing* 9(6):315-23, November/December 1983.

Index

i refers to an illustration; t refers to a table

i refers to an illustration; t refers to a table

i refers to an illustration; t refers to a table

i refers to an illustration; t refers to a table

i refers to an illustration; t refers to a table

i refers to an illustration; t refers to a table

Notes

Notes

Notes